THE CLINICIAN'S HANDBOOK ON
MEASUREMENT-BASED CARE

The How,
The What, and
The Why Bother

Antoinette Giedzinska, Ph.D.
Director of the Research Institute,
Cumberland Heights Foundation,
Nashville, Tennessee

Aaron R. Wilson, M.D.
Chief Medical Officer,
Sonora Behavioral Health Hospital (Acadia Healthcare),
Cornerstone Behavioral Health El Dorado,
Cottonwood Tucson, and Sabino Recovery, Tucson;
Assistant Clinical Professor of Psychiatry,
Creighton University School of Medicine,
Phoenix, Arizona

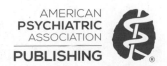
AMERICAN
PSYCHIATRIC
ASSOCIATION
PUBLISHING

If you wish to buy 50 or more copies of the same title, please go to www.appi.org/specialdiscounts for more information.

Copyright © 2023 American Psychiatric Association Publishing

ALL RIGHTS RESERVED

First Edition

Manufactured in the United States of America on acid-free paper
26 25 24 23 22   5 4 3 2 1

American Psychiatric Association Publishing
800 Maine Avenue SW, Suite 900
Washington, DC 20024-2812
www.appi.org

Library of Congress Cataloging-in-Publication Data
A CIP record is available from the Library of Congress.

British Library Cataloguing in Publication Data
A CIP record is available from the British Library.

Contents

PART I
The WHY
*What Is Measurement-Based Care, and
Why Should You Bother?*

PART II
The HOW
The "Methods" in Measurement-Based Care

Foreword

T_{HIS} book is a must read for all behavioral health care and human services clinicians and leaders who aspire to lead their practice and organization into a successful and prosperous future. It provides the "how to" information for using measurement-based care (MBC), the critical component to delivering high-quality, high-value care, treatment, and services .

The use of MBC in behavioral health care and human services will likely have the greatest impact on moving this industry forward now and in the future. In seeking parity in access to health care resources, behavioral health care and human services clinicians and organizations must demonstrate measurable outcomes for the care, treatment, and services they provide to the individuals they serve. The medical health care sector has long provided clinical data to demonstrate the degree to which individuals stabilize or improve from the care delivered, thus showing measurable value for the resources used to deliver care. Behavioral health care and human services organizations have not done the same and therefore have struggled to achieve parity with payers, regulators, patients, and other important stakeholders. In 2018, seeking to help move the field forward, the Joint Commission (TJC) Behavioral Health Care and Human Services accreditation program introduced a standard requiring all of its accredited organizations to use MBC in the delivery of care, treatment, and services to the individuals they serve, making TJC the only accreditor to require its use.

As the executive director of the Behavioral Health Care and Human Services program at TJC, I knew this change represented an immense step forward for the clinicians and organizations currently accredited and those seeking accreditation. As a result, we needed to collaborate with innovative leaders who have effectively implemented MBC in order to help these organizations move forward. Dr. Giedzinska was recommended to me as a leader who had embraced MBC and was using it effectively within her organization, Sierra Tucson. To that end, Dr. Giedzinska has been a valued collaborator in our endeavor to move the use of MBC forward. She has shared her organization's journey in implementing MBC with our accredited organizations and those seeking accreditation. She has demonstrated an in-depth knowledge of MBC, the benefits of its use, how to implement it in an organization effectively, and how to use data from MBC throughout the course of care and to improve the services offered by her organization to the entire population it serves. By way of this book, she is now sharing this valuable information with the industry at large.

Many behavioral health care and human services clinicians and organizations struggle to get started with utilizing MBC. It is important for them to understand the return on investment for using MBC in terms of the improvements in the clinical outcomes of the individuals they serve; overall improvements in the quality and safety of the care, treatment, and services provided; and recognition from external parties such as regulators, payers, and associations. Through this book, the authors demonstrate that these goals can be achieved through the use of MBC.

In this book, Dr. Giedzinska utilizes her advanced training and extensive experience in clinical psychology and program leadership to guide readers through the journey of embracing MBC in a practical manner. She helps them overcome the fear of embarking on this new journey by breaking it into steps that are easy to understand and implement. She presents a compelling reason to use MBC, in partnership with the individual served, to improve the therapeutic alliance, reinforce patient progress, and improve clinical outcomes. Furthermore, she demonstrates that aggregating the data from the population served aids in improving program fidelity, demonstrates value to third parties, and improves the overall quality and safety of the services provided to all the individuals served by the clinician or organization.

Her views in this book on the importance of MBC and her practical tips on implementation and use of the data will guide the behavioral health care and human services industry and all the individuals it serves.

Julia S. Finken, R.N., B.S.N., M.B.A., CPHQ, CLSSMBB
Executive Director,
Behavioral Health Care and Human Services,
The Joint Commission,
Oakbrook Terrace, Illinois

Preface

MEASUREMENT-BASED care (MBC). Chances are, if you are reading this right now, you are considering how to implement this process into your clinical practice. The good news: you have opened the right book. The not-so-good news: there is a bit of work ahead of you (or your team) to put this process into practice, but those efforts are worthwhile. There is a lot of goodness in implementing MBC, and not only for your patients but also for you and your clinical practice. In fact, implementing MBC practices into mental health treatment may be very good for our industry overall.

If you are like us, you are very busy and probably have already advanced through to some of the chapters in this book to check out the specific sections relevant to you. That's great, but we ask that you first read Section I before diving in to start implementing the hands-on approaches offered in the rest of this book. Section I sets the stage and foundation for the "WHAT", the "WHY," and the "HOW" of MBC. As a busy clinician, familiarizing yourself with this content is important because if you cannot justify why on Earth you are spending all this extra time and resources to measure your patient's mental health progress, chances are you will not stick with these methods. And you will want to stick with them, because there are more benefits to integrating MBC into your practice than there are for NOT integrating it into your practice.

Before you begin, it is important to understand some of the potential barriers—largely based on misconceptions—that require consideration, which Section I outlines. One of these is the age-old debate between clinical and actuarial judgment. In mental health patient-centered care, these two aspects serve patients better when they are integrated rather than viewed as contentious adversaries. Another potential barrier to implementation is the understandable fear surrounding the "punitive" nature that patient-reported progress data may have on one's clinical competence. This is largely a myth worth demystifying. Practice fidelity is a reality to which all of us must hold ourselves accountable, and MBC processes can actually serve as the foundation on which therapeutic practice fidelity rests. Have you ever met a mental health practitioner who did therapeutic clinical work for any reason other than the desire to help reduce patients' suffering? Not likely. Therefore, we want our approaches to work, and additional information that informs us about our patients' mental health progress is something clinicians should embrace rather than fear. MBC is one of those methods that will help you help others, and better than you ever thought possible.

The benefits of MBC far outweigh any barriers, in our opinion. For the past 20 years, numerous empirical studies have demonstrated the positive impact that MBC has had on therapeutic success. There is collective agreement that when mental health clinicians review the self-reported data with their patients, whether as the initial assessment of the patient's psychological profile or as the mid-treatment review of the patient's therapeutic progress, the therapeutic alliance and rapport are strengthened as a result. Patients' clinical presentation is supported by the data, which appears to have a validating effect—and we know the therapeutic power that validating patients can have. When patients are able to discuss these data with their clinician, that important need to be heard and understood is expanded dimensionally. For instance, discussing self-reported data epitomizes patient-centered care by strengthening collaborative treatment decision-making and ultimately enhancing personalized treatment plans. Consider thus how this process would promote treatment compliance; one of the most important findings from implementing MBC throughout treatment is its ability to prevent treatment failure by catching patients who would otherwise imperceptibly "fall through the cracks."

Using psychometric data in this manner becomes one of your most powerful clinical tools. Trust us on this: Once you overcome bias, fears, or even challenges to your ego (yes, we all know at least one clinician among us with "clinical pride") and integrate the methods outlined in this book, your clinical practice will be more effective, your patients will show better treatment responses, and you, yourself, will likely have greater job satisfaction.

Antoinette Giedzinska, Ph.D.
Aaron R. Wilson, M.D.

PART I

The WHY

What Is Measurement-Based Care, and Why Should You Bother?

Chapter
01

What Is Measurement-Based Care?

Iterations of Outcomes Measurement

Typical of many of our colleagues working busily in their own corners of the clinical and academic world, the designation for the process of measuring mental health treatment progress and treatment outcomes has varied over the past years, taking on such iterations as measurement-based care (MBC; Scott and Lewis 2015), routine outcomes monitoring (Ellwood 1988), progress monitoring (Goodman et al. 2013), and concurrent recovery monitoring (McLellan et al. 2005), just to name a few. Since 1998, the Commission on Accreditation of Rehabilitation Facilities (CARF; 2017) has required its facilities to implement programs of outcomes management to assess patients, track progress, and report outcomes, yet much of the momentum toward implementing this practice into mental health is due to the powerful policy issue brief published by the Kennedy Forum in 2015 (Fortney et al. 2015). This report outlined the importance of adding psychometric scales to enhance treatment decision-making and treatment plan alterations, achieve deeper therapeutic alliance, and prevent treatment failure. In January 2018, The Joint Commission published the revision to its Outcome Measures Standard CTS 03.01.09 requiring mental health accredited facilities to implement the use of valid psychometric scales. The revision's directive is not only to gauge treatment progress but also to show that treatment plans are modified based in part on a review of patient reports from those psychometric scales.

The term *measurement-based care* captures the essence of using psychometric scales as tools to enhance understanding of mental health issues and to support the clinical process; it is therefore our chosen designation and is used as such throughout this book. Variations of published designations aside, there is also the issue of ubiquitously agreed-upon accepted definitions for MBC. For instance, Scott and Lewis (2015) defined MBC as "the practice of basing clinical care on patient data collected throughout treatment" (p. 49), whereas Lewis et al. (2019) specified "the systematic evaluation of patient symptoms before or during each clinical encounter to inform behavioral health treatment" (p. 324). Fortney et al. (2017) defined MBC as entailing "the systematic administration of symptom rating scales to use the results to drive clinical decision making at the level of the individual patient" (p. 180), and Kearney et al. (2015) stated that MBC is "the systematic collection of data to monitor treatment progress, assess outcomes, and guide treatment decisions, from initial screening to completion of care" (p. 213). The overlapping consensus is that some form of quantifiable evaluation of mental health symptoms should be collected and used to *inform treatment*; disparities appear to primarily exist in the methods of MBC.

Our Definition

Having implemented MBC practice for several years now, we prefer the definition put forth by Wray et al. (2018) because it captures the essence of how we use MBC. The use of MBC can be expanded beyond this definition to include utilizing the initial administration of psychometric testing to support the clinical diagnostic formulation. A working diagnostic hypothesis can be substantiated by reviewing self-reported psychometric data and discussing those findings directly with the patient. Data from "pre" treatment measures serve more in this instance than simply providing a baseline to which repeated administration of subsequent measures throughout the treatment trajectory will be compared.

As providers of mental health treatment, we have also found it invaluable to aggregate the data to assess program fidelity. All clinicians, either in private practice, group practice, or larger treatment facilities, are ethically obligated to ensure that they are providing best practices. How will you really know the effectiveness of your treatment process or clinical program without having collected systematic data across patient populations and over time? We all love "testimonials," and many of us share these on our practice brochures and websites, but to truly put money where your mouth is, we recommend backing up those testimonials with honest, clean, aggregated data. If you are part of an accredited practice, The Joint Commission and CARF require it. If you are on insurance panels, third-party payers may request it.

Therefore, MBC becomes much more than tossing in a few valid psychometric scales as part of your practice; *it is a system of measuring patient progress at the individual level and of measuring program fidelity at the systemic level.*

As authors, we now join our professional colleagues by contributing to the already existing collection of MBC definitions. Our definition underscores the framework for methods outlined in this book:

> Measurement-based care is the systematic collection of individual data acquired at initial screening, at various identified times during treatment, and at completion of care. Its primary function is to serve as a clinical tool to support clinical practice in order to substantiate diagnostic formulation, guide treatment decisions, monitor treatment progress, and evaluate treatment outcomes at the individual level. Its secondary function is to evaluate program fidelity in aggregate form as a method of quality assurance to evaluate treatment effectiveness, analyze outcomes, understand predictors of patient progress, and determine factors toward treatment improvement.

Using Measures to Guide Clinical Practice and Improve Treatment Response

What's Not to Love?
Benefits of Integrating Measurement-Based Care Into Your Clinical Practice

Clinical psychologists have long known that psychometric evaluation augments clinical practice by clarifying symptom presentation, differentiating diagnoses, and deepening understanding of the clinical profile. Using psychometric data to yield deeper understanding about a patient's psychological profile through subsequent clinical feedback serves to benefit both clinician and patient alike. The practice of measurement-based care (MBC) comprises the initial screening for this purpose, and when measures are administered at various times throughout treatment to gauge and openly discuss treatment progress as part of the therapeutic hour, patient benefits appear to take on greater therapeutic meaning. This section outlines some of the established benefits of integrating MBC into clinical practice. These benefits might be considered "mechanisms of success" because they are, for all intents and purposes, both secondary gains and mediators of the MBC feedback loop. Each of these is summarized here.

Therapeutic Alliance

Miller et al. (2006), in their landmark study to determine the utility of feedback-informed treatment using pre- and post-encounter four-item scales, identified that through this early method of MBC, study participants reported improved therapeutic alliance and treatment satisfaction from discussing their survey responses with their therapists as part of the clinical process. The authors noted that therapist–patient feedback regarding alliance and progress was associated with significant improvements in both patient retention and treatment outcomes. This method of feedback-informed treatment, when reformulated in other studies, demonstrated that patients who engaged in measurement-based progress feedback found their therapists to be more empathetic and better listeners compared with those who did not (Guo et al. 2015; Shimokawa et al. 2010). In a qualitative study assessing 34 primary care clinics, Dowrick et al. (2009) noted that depressed patients were very receptive to symptom rating scales and that the scales improved communication between patient and provider. Most patients considered that discussing data during therapy was an example of providers "taking their mental health problems seriously."

The mechanisms by which MBC strengthens therapeutic alliance can be attributed to satiating the basic human need for heartfelt connectedness (Frank and Frank 1991). Patients' feelings of trust and engagement are increased when an attentive clinician reviews their progress data by describing their concerns and using that information in a meaningful way to help them. Fortney et al. (2017) proposed that MBC has the potential to enhance the therapeutic relationship between patient and provider, leading to a more informed and engaged patient who can participate meaningfully in shared decision-making. Therapy patients need to feel heard and want to have a connection with their clinician. Discussing therapeutic progress, whether to identify improvement or worsening, opens up a direct opportunity of communication, connectedness, and collaboration.

Therapeutic Compliance

Noncompliance is a well-documented problem in all fields of medicine, including psychiatry and psychotherapy practices (Farooq and Naeem 2014). Noncompliance has a major impact on the success of treatment; if patients do not adhere to their treatment plan faithfully, even the most exemplary evidence-based treatment approaches will not yield the intended beneficial outcomes. Therapeutic compliance includes patient compliance not only with medication but also with diet, exercise, or lifestyle changes (Jin et al. 2008). Noncompliance is estimated to be more than 75% for short-term psychotherapy and nearly 50% for long-term medication therapies (Semahegn et al. 2018) and is a legitimate concern for those of us in the helping professions.

Patient factors such as motivational issues or negative attitudes toward therapy are commonly perceived as contributing most often to noncompliance. Several studies have shown that patients' negative attitudes toward therapy are associated with their level of treatment compliance (Jette et al. 1998; Kilbourne et al. 2005; Melamed and Szor 1999; Sirey et al. 2001). Those who evince low motivation to change also have been shown to have poor compliance (Spikmans et al. 2003); motivation can be negatively impacted by depression, which can then serve as a double-edged sword when clinicians attempt to keep this patient population engaged during therapy (Melamed and Szor 1999).

Patient factors alone are not entirely responsible for noncompliance. The therapeutic relationship also is a strong factor (Gonzalez et al. 2005; Löffler et al. 2003; Moore et al. 2004). A healthy relationship is based on patients' trust in their clinician and a feeling that their provider is empathetic (Moore et al. 2004). Communication between therapist and patient also has been shown to correlate directly with patient compliance behaviors (Jin et al. 2008).

If there were a magic wand to dispel noncompliance in patients, we would have all bought one by now. Clearly, there is no simple solution; patients are people, and people, whether seeking mental health treatment or not, tend to bustle with complexities. Implementation of MBC into the psychotherapeutic process has shown to reduce the likelihood of noncompliance for the reasons outlined earlier. In their review article describing MBC through the Treatment Outcome Package, Youn et al. (2012) observed the potential for secondary gains from receiving feedback-informed care. One of those gains was patients having a greater ability to detect slight improvement as a direct result of receiving progress feedback. As a result, these patients had greater motivation and expressed more hope because they were making "recognizable progress." Recognizing progress by observing even the slightest change in data points can serve to validate and substantiate patients' experience and help them trust the therapeutic process. Feeling hopeful about their treatment plan and progress is a likely contributing factor in patients continuing or complying with treatment.

In a quasi-experimental study assessing the effects of MBC, Eisen et al. (2000) observed that patients who discussed their symptom rating scales with their therapists were likely to be more active in the treatment process. Moreover, reviewing progress data allowed for deeper understanding and clarification, which in turn created a format for better doctor–patient communication. In several review articles (Fortney et al. 2017; Lambert 2017; Lewis et al. 2019), it has been consistently noted that enhanced therapeutic engagement and hopefulness and improved communication with clinicians are the direct results of receiving MBC. To abate noncompliance, clinicians must focus on building healthy relationships with their patients to foster the patients' involvement in designing the treatment plan (Gonzalez et al. 2005; Vlasnik et al. 2005) and must offer emotional support and reassurance while engaging patients in the care plan (Jin et al. 2008). What better way to accomplish these objectives than through the additional implementation of MBC?

Patient Insight

The essence of insight comprises both knowledge and understanding derived from an "inward sight" (Shelley 1821), and its diminishment is often associated with many psychiatric disorders. To garner insight is thought to be primarily a function of our frontal lobe executive functioning networks. According to Rubin and Zorumski (2016), higher-order brain abilities—and thus insight—are often dysfunctional in most psychiatric disorders.

In 2009, the Group for the Advancement of Psychiatry published a call to action to implement MBC into clinical practice. They stipulated that when patients regularly complete self-reported rating scales as part of the therapeutic process, they are likely to become more knowledgeable about their disorders, attuned to the fluctuation of their symptoms over time, and cognizant of the warning signs of relapse or reoccurrence (Valenstein et al. 2009). A possible function of MBC is that the repeated behavior to review symptom rating scales likely enhances patients' ability to better recognize their own psychological state. Fortney et al. (2017) suggested that MBC enhances the progress of insight quicker than psychotherapy alone.

Insight alone may not be an essential requirement for psychotherapy to be effective, but it certainly can precipitate learned responses associated with behavioral change or cognitive shifts. Effective psychotherapy engenders learning and, thus, change. Self-awareness or insight may be a factor that sustains successful long-term recovery (Moeller and Goldstein 2014) as well as an indicator of therapeutic growth and recovery.

Preventing Treatment Failure

Perhaps one of the most compelling benefits of MBC is its function to prevent treatment failure. Many well-designed studies, theoretical papers, and review articles have been dedicated to this topic. Based on the need to compensate for clinical judgment inaccuracies, the early research led by Michael Lambert and Scott Miller consistently demonstrated that feedback-informed psychotherapy outperformed treatment as usual with respect to enhanced therapeutic alliance (Miller et al. 2006), faster symptom improvement (Bickman et al. 2011), better overall outcomes (Lambert 2017; Whipple et al. 2003), and, most importantly, identifying patients who were *not* improving as expected in therapy *well in advance of treatment completion* (Lambert 2007, 2017; Lewis et al. 2019). These authors and others collectively advised that clinical deterioration can be prevented as a result of monitoring therapeutic progress through feedback-informed care.

The goal of MBC is to substantiate the status of therapeutic progress. As part of feedback-informed care, the comparison between current status and previous status provides the opportunity to celebrate positive growth, recognize clinical inertia, or identify therapeutic deterioration. In all three conditions, discussing reported progress provided by psychometric measures is essential to further understand your patient, explore potential alterations to the treatment plan to best serve the patient's needs (Lambert et al. 2003; Morris and Trivedi 2011), and improve the therapeutic relationship or process through continued support and validation. This is the essence of MBC, and it further underscores clinical best practices. In an article in *World Psychiatry*, Kilbourne et al. (2018) advocated for meaningful improvement in the quality of mental health services universally, and one of their recommendations was adopting routinized MBC to provide a consistent quality of care and improve patient outcomes.

Why MBC is touted as critical to capturing treatment failure is largely due to the shortcomings of clinical judgment in accurately identifying patients who are not progressing over the course of treatment or those who ultimately deteriorate without detection upon discharge (Lambert 2017). Psychotherapy comprises art, craft, science, and a great amount of humanity, epitomizing humans helping humans. Because of the complexities of human nature, it is not surprising that inaccuracies in judgment occur. According to Lambert (2017), clinicians have "very little control over the patients' life circumstances and personal characteristics" (p. 82), which influences patients' response to treatment. Whether influenced by self-assessment bias, an overly optimistic attitude about their own therapeutic skill set, or simply their humanness, the fact remains that clinicians do not always accurately grasp the progress of their patients.

Failure to predict treatment failure is not an inconsequential occurrence. It has been estimated that 50% of patients fail to improve after receiving psychotherapy (Miller 2015). Per 2017 statistics from the Substance Abuse and Mental Health Services Administration (2018), more than 46 million Americans have some type of psychiatric disorder, with an estimated 20 million of those seeking mental health treatment. Therefore, the 10 million individuals who do not benefit from psychotherapy treatment should be concerning. Curiously, Walfish et al. (2012) reported that when clinicians were queried about their therapeutic outcomes, they reported on average a 77% success rate and an even lower 4% perceived failure rate. You do the math. Clinical perception of failure is a far cry from national estimated patient failure rates.

Adding an objective psychometric process to clinical practice essentially supplements clinical judgment, boosting the clinician's perception of progress and, more importantly, buoying the patient. Lambert (2017) referred to this as the "signal alarm system." MBC essentially helps clinicians become aware of negative change, thereby providing opportunities to explore issues that their current treatment plan is not supporting. Changes to treatment can be addressed and proceeded. This function is fundamental to The Joint Commission's 2018 mandate for MBC implementation. The mandate to Outcome Measures Standard CTS 03.01.09 was based on the compelling, consistent outcomes of research demonstrating that MBC does, in fact, catch patients before or when they fall through the proverbial cracks.

What's Holding You Back?
Challenging Biases and Reframing Misconceptions About Psychometric Measures

The benefits of implementing MBC into your clinical practice outweigh any of the challenges of launching and maintaining such a program. Before we consider the ways in which MBC can guide your practice and enhance your patients' response to treatment, it is important to address the biases against and misconceptions about the psychometric tests and standardized procedures surrounding psychometric administration. Maybe you hold some of these biases yourself, and maybe you do not; but it is likely that a few of these beliefs are deeply ingrained in the clinical schemata of many of your trusted colleagues. Addressing attitudes and concerns about psychological testing is critical to implementing a successful MBC program.

Bias #1: Self-Assessment Bias

Self-assessment bias—or, "my clinical judgment is just fine, thank you very much. I don't need to bother using some psychiatric symptom scale to help me do my job"—may be one of those taboo dinner topics to avoid, akin to politics and religion.

Self-assessment bias among mental health clinicians is a real thing; Walfish et al. (2012) observed that among 129 mental health clinicians, more than half overestimated their clinical successes while underestimating their clinical failures. According to Dunning et al. (2004), such estimates are statistically impossible. Others also have reported findings of clinicians incorrectly predicting successful therapeutic improvement in their patients (Boswell et al. 2015; Sapyta et al. 2005) or, worse, incorrectly predicting treatment deterioration (Hannan et al. 2005; Hatfield et al. 2010). When patients plateau—or "clinical inertia" develops—clinical detection rates are shown to be even worse (Hannan et al. 2005; Henke et al. 2009). (See "Preventing Treatment Failure" section earlier in this chapter for additional discussion.)

The clinical challenges to systematically recognizing clinical inertia or treatment deterioration are an inconvenient truth and a significant concern in psychotherapy. Lambert (2017) cautioned that "failure to recognize that a patient is not responding to treatment is a serious problem in routine care and one that appears to be made worse by the clinicians' confidence in their clinical judgment and unique healing gifts" (p. 82). A viable solution to bias is to implement MBC methods to monitor treatment response. Zimmerman and McGlinchey (2008) suggested that symptom rating scales can alert clinicians when patients develop treatment inertia or begin to deteriorate, which may then prompt discussion about changing the treatment plan. Augmenting clinical judgment with objective self-report data can bolster confidence in assessing patient progress and can detect—and thus avoid—treatment failure.

Bias #2: Self-Report Response Bias

Self-report symptom scales are prone to response bias and therefore provide questionable or limited clinical information. One of the major threats to validity in behavioral science and epidemiological research is the possibility of self-report response bias. Whether conducting an interview or administering a survey, inaccurate reporting is often a potential risk. The degree of honesty with which patients answer survey questions is a valid concern, and biases can range from social desirability to recall bias, ultimately negatively impacting data (Althubaiti 2016). When self-report data are properly managed, however, they can provide a greater range of information than many other forms of data collection instruments (Zhu et al. 1999).

Response bias is not specific to psychometric testing; it is also a threat to the validity of the clinical interview. During intake or even during the therapeutic hour, there is always the risk that patients will discuss their symptoms in the way they think you want to hear. As clinicians, we rely on patient dialogue and self-report as part of the therapeutic process. Thus, we assume that patients enlist our help because they genuinely want to reduce their suffering and that they will approach any self-report symptom scale or clinical interview with honest disclosure. It is prudent to approach your MBC program with the full knowledge that the information obtained, either through self-report survey or clinical interview, may be biased. Despite these risks, self-report is the essence of effective psychotherapy, and the manner in which we address reported biases through talk therapy is the same manner in which we address it through MBC.

Misconception #1: MBC Is Time Consuming and Expensive

Concerns about the time and financial costs of MBC primarily arise from misconceptions by uninitiated clinicians who quickly assume there is little variation to MBC implementation. The essence of this book is to provide you with the steps for implementing the most effective method of MBC to support your practice, considering your skill sets while respecting the routine pragmatic factors and constraints of running a clinical practice. According to Fortney et al. (2017), factors such as additional paperwork, time, and lack of personnel are the reasons clinicians do not implement MBC. Lucock et al. (2015) reported that barriers in implementing MBC included practical issues of time burden, having to prepare reports to multiple stakeholders, and staff support. They also identified therapist fear and mistrust about MBC as problematic to implementation (see "Bias #1" and "Bias #2" sections earlier).

Time concerns are not reserved only for clinicians; patients also play a key role in MBC as the individuals who complete the assessments. Symptom severity may inversely impact patients' ability to complete symptom scales (de Jong et al. 2018), especially after intense therapeutic sessions (Lucock et al. 2015). Nevertheless, most patients find that the benefits of receiving MBC feedback outweigh the burdens of completing psychological scales (Fortney et al. 2017; Lambert 2007; Lucock et al. 2015; Zimmerman and McGlinchey 2008). In fact, during focus group debriefings, Lucock et al. (2015) learned that study participants not only reported notable benefit from MBC but also recommended that their therapists review MBC progress data as part of the therapeutic process.

Psychiatric symptom measures used for MBC do not have to be large, all-encompassing, time-consuming, expensive batteries. In fact, measures are plentiful and range from very brief and free to substantial and expensive. Zimmerman and McGlinchey (2008) advised that "scales should be brief, ideally taking no more than 2–3 minutes to complete, so that upon repeated administration at follow-up visits, patients are not inconvenienced by the need to come for their appointment 10–15 minutes early in order to complete the measure" (p. 125). A win-win is possible. Moreover, the psychological scales you choose should streamline your practice and yield more time in the therapy hour for deeper clinical work—a third "win." We have known several talented clinicians who began their therapeutic hour perfunctorily reviewing a symptom checklist with their patients. Imagine that for a moment. Although the spirit of compassion and caring is evident in this process, precious time for developing alliance and working toward therapeutic depth is instead spent reviewing a psychiatric symptom shopping list. Having patients complete a pre-session assessment and making these data immediately available frees you to hone right in on the issue(s) reported and frees your patients from interminable interviews. The return for that little extra time needed to complete and score an assessment may be worth the effort.

Dare we mention a potential fourth "win"? Several recent publications and presentations have offered compelling justification that managed care should implement reimbursement for MBC practices just as it does for other medical assessments (Fortney et al. 2015, 2017; Powell et al. 2019). Laboratory tests, biometric measurements, and diagnostic screenings (e.g., X-ray, MRI) used to diagnose illness and gauge recovery are commonly covered by managed care.

MBC is analogous to these acceptable practices of symptom progress monitoring. Furthermore, peer-reviewed studies have shown that repeated psychological screening for mental health patients leads to substantially improved outcomes (Fortney et al. 2017) and reduced costs (Powell et al. 2019). Guo et al. (2015) observed that depressed patients receiving MBC evinced significantly greater treatment response and remission in comparison with those in the "treatment as usual" condition. Current Procedural Terminology (CPT) codes already exist for a number of psychometric assessments used for diagnostic purposes, and others appear potentially applicable for progress monitoring and outcomes assessment associated with MBC practices. The caveat is that although, in theory, CPT codes may cover the cost of MBC, their frequency of use and the number of psychiatric symptom scales administered may be limited (Powell et al. 2019). At present, reimbursement policies lack uniformity, and insurance companies trail behind in adopting MBC despite multiple research studies showing that standardized measures must be administered frequently to properly guide treatment decisions and improve outcomes (Fortney et al. 2015). Table 2–1 lists the current CPT codes that may be assigned for MBC reimbursement at this time.

The current state of managed care's relationship with MBC is best understood as the growing pains associated with actively traversing a paradigm shift rather than proving the assumption that insurance companies are refusing to listen. But we do have an uphill battle. Raney et al. (2017) sagaciously quipped that the payer's perspective is that "behavioral health is a black hole: we pour money into it and we don't get anything in return"

TABLE 2–1.   **Current Procedural Terminology codes likely to be used for measurement-based care reimbursement**

Code	Description
96127	Brief emotional/behavioral assessment (e.g., depression inventory, ADHD scale, with scoring and documentation, per standardized instrument)
96146	Psychological or neuropsychological test administration (with single automated, standardized instrument via electronic platform, with automated result only)
96136	Psychological or neuropsychological test administration and scoring by physician or other qualified health care professional (two or more tests, any method; up to first 30 minutes)
96138	Psychological or neuropsychological test administration and scoring by technician (two or more tests, any method; up to first 30 minutes)

(p. 7). This stance is supported by a history of limited success in the behavioral health care industry. The operative word here is *history*. As more studies add to the growing body of MBC evidence and more clinicians employ MBC in their practices (and use their data to substantiate treatment success), chances are that managed care's stance will collectively shift toward seeing behavioral health in a positive light and thus lead to better coverage.

Misconception #2: MBC Is Outcomes Research

The perception of MBC as outcomes research might be described as "I'm a clinician, not a researcher; implementing measurement-based care requires advanced understanding of research design and statistics." Even if this sentiment is not directly articulated, it may be seen in the glazed eyes of our clinical colleagues in response to the sheer mention of MBC. Differentiating the nuances between MBC and outcomes research is fundamental to successfully implement MBC. Until recently, designations such as "outcomes research" or "mental health outcomes" have been widely used in social media and peer-reviewed literature to include behavioral health treatment effectiveness along with traditional practice outcomes. Historically, outcomes research has been the jurisdiction of clinical efficacy studies and behavioral health science, which certainly does require special research design skill sets.

However, MBC is different. First, it is *not* outcomes research. It can incorporate psychotherapy outcomes, but from a *clinical therapeutic standpoint at the individual level*. Its use of symptom rating scales to monitor therapeutic progress throughout treatment is fundamental, so evaluating outcomes is only one aspect. Second, outcomes research in general requires study designs to assess treatment efficacy or effectiveness. It uses research methods as the framework within which participants are assigned to various treatment conditions for which controlling various factors or conditions is necessary. It involves consent forms, institutional review boards, sample size considerations, and—dare we say it—statistics. This is not MBC. MBC is accomplished in the naturalistic setting: the clinic. Standardizing the methods with which you assess your patients is highly recommended (and is covered in Section II of this book), but these methods are for ascertaining that patients are benefiting from the most effective mental health treatment possible. Therefore, the use of psychological scales in MBC is *clinical*, specifically for the purpose of enhancing treatment, engendering treatment alliance, and deepening clinical understanding.

Aggregating MBC data for evaluating a treatment program is discussed in greater detail in Section IV of this book; quality assurance evaluation differs from outcomes research in many ways, and greater clarification about these distinctions is needed. However, many readers will likely only use MBC at the individual level, and if this describes you, then you can breathe a sigh of relief and read only what is applicable to your own practice, outlined in Sections II and III.

Misconception #3: Only Psychologists Can Administer Psychological Testing

Historically speaking, "psychological" testing in the clinical process falls under the authority of professional psychologists. Regardless, any measure used to assess an attribute or characteristic, or even to predict an outcome, can be considered a psychological test. This includes not only the expected psychological batteries to assess intelligence, aptitude, and personality but also vocational testing, symptom scales, quality-of-life functioning, and even the love-language tests found in beauty magazines. Undoubtedly, the latter measures are not always administered under the watchful eye of a psychologist.

Despite the loose demarcations, the *Standards for Educational and Psychological Testing* (American Educational Research Association et al. 2014) stipulate that psychologists are the clinicians trained to understand psychometric rigor as it relates to testing theory, test development, and assessing whether tests meet these standards to qualify their usefulness. Psychologists are also uniquely trained and qualified to conduct assessments within the boundaries of their competence. It is thus important to distinguish between *assessment* and *testing* because psychological assessment differs significantly from psychological testing. There is no loose demarcation here, according to the American Psychological Association (2010). The expertise to respond to a mental health referral with the appropriate selection of tests, clinical interviews, medical records, and collateral information relies squarely on the competence of the psychologist. This multifaceted approach is what constitutes psychological assessment. Psychological tests are just one element of the larger integrated assessment.

Therefore, which mental health professionals can obtain and use what appears to be an endless array of psychological scales? The actual answer is not clear. Two of the main psychological testing publishers, Pearson and Psychological Assessment Resources, uphold certification requirements limiting the use and purchase of their tests. These qualification policies range from Qualification Level A (no special qualifications needed) to Qualification Level C (appropriate doctoral degree, licensure, or certification required). Nevertheless, a vast collection of psychometrically sound mental health measures is also available for free and often found in the public domain. Use of these symptom scales and quality-of-life measures are typically not limited to use only by licensed psychologists; most can be obtained and used by non-psychologist clinicians as well. In Section III, we review the distinguishing levels of psychological testing, use permission, and psychometrics to further bolster your appreciation and understanding so that you can make educated decisions when choosing MBC scales.

Misconception #4: Progress Evaluation That Indicates Deterioration Means I Have Failed

The signal alarm system of MBC is designed to work *with* providers, not against them. One of the main purposes of MBC is to identify treatment deterioration or clinical inertia *before* it becomes official treatment failure. Several years ago, when discussing the goodness of implementing MBC at a professional conference, an audience member innocently asked, "But what if the data show our programs are not successful?" Our answer? "We learn from it." It was clear that a difference in perspective was evident. On the one hand, most marketing outreach would want to "measure to impress," and on the other, quality assurance guides us to "measure to improve." Considering how your core values interface with MBC is a worthwhile exercise and a likely side effect of reading this book.

As clinical professionals, proper and consistent evaluation is essential to our personal growth; indirectly, MBC may serve as a clinical evaluation of our overall effectiveness. Therefore, fear of failure may be a formidable barrier to implementing a system that will alert you to the possibility of treatment failure. However, if you are evaluating treatment progress and discussing these findings with your patients in earnest, then you will likely not be blindsided by therapeutic deterioration. This is the goodness of MBC. Understandably, we must take inventory of our own personal clinical insecurities while holding ourselves accountable for delivering treatment in the manner we intend to practice it. You do this work because you want to help others; therefore, you want your therapy to work. It bears repeating that the signal alarm system of MBC is designed to work with you, not against you.

Summary

Quite simply, progress data are the pepper to the salt of psychotherapy. When used clinically, data from measures do more than simply "quantify" MBC; *good data help tell the story of therapeutic healing*. Although data are inherently scientific, the tangibility of presenting and discussing data can be truly magical when it promotes the noteworthy "A-ha!" moment of psychological insight or therapeutic hope. The upfront time and effort you put into developing and implementing MBC are worthy endeavors indeed because, when integrated into clinical process, it can fortify your overall practice and programming.

PART II

The HOW

The "Methods" in Measurement-Based Care

Chapter 03

Getting Started

THE field of measurement-based care (MBC) has seen exponential growth since the mandate set forth by the Kennedy Forum in 2015. Although it was a game-changing initiative toward the betterment of the behavioral health industry, the breeze of MBC's acceleration inevitably has been felt throughout the industry, leaving many clinicians in its wake, likely confused and a bit lost on how to get started with implementing MBC into their practice.

Not surprisingly, a number of innovative online platforms are available to offer MBC services, for a fee. At the time of this writing, more than 10 cloud-based businesses have been launched. Partnering with an online firm may be the best decision for many busy clinical practices, but before considering this option, you should establish clear practice guidelines regarding the utility of MBC, its methods, and how best to implement it into your practice. This will help you determine which online platform best aligns with your practice mission. The other, likely less expensive option is to implement a do-it-yourself (DIY) approach. Regardless of which option you choose, one of the aims of this book is to provide the foundations of MBC so that any independent practitioner or larger clinical practice will be informed and prepared to incorporate MBC into their unique practice model.

The purpose of Part II is to offer a basic introduction to the operations of MBC and explain how to implement valid assessment methods. A sustainable MBC program will entail much more than administering symptoms scales. It is a transdisciplinary process that weaves the predictable structure of scientific methodology into the nuanced practice of psychotherapy. Exploring and then implementing certain research methods, such as operationalizing, determining test validity, and structuring reliable administration, is the backbone of a successful MBC practice.

Defining the Why and the Art of Operationalization

Operationalization is basically a process to objectively define a concept or construct in a way that it can be measured (Emilio 2003). It is usually one of the first important steps necessary for conducting meaningful behavioral health research; defining variables into objective measurable constructs is key to study construction. Although MBC is advocated to augment the *clinical* process, at its foundation it is a data collection method and thus necessitates following certain accepted research practices. The first step to routinizing MBC so that it synergizes with a clinical practice or therapeutic program is to operationally define the practice mission, aims, and therapeutic orientation.

Deconstructing your practice mission and therapeutic orientation will provide the context to guide interpretation of therapeutic progress and outcomes. Good data tell the story of the therapeutic trajectory; therefore, the stage on which therapy is conducted must be defined for meaningful MBC. Reporting a decrease in psychiatric symptoms without including the context in which that psychotherapeutic effect took place yields limited clarity about the mechanisms of change. For example, how a cognitive-behavioral therapy (CBT) practitioner views progress in depression may differ from how an emotion-focused provider considers progress. In CBT, therapeutic progress may be measured by a change in distorted perceptions defined by strongly held core beliefs or unrealistic expectations of self and others (Beck 2011). Measuring a reduction in depression in this case would involve observing a reduction in harmful thoughts or a demonstrated ability to challenge negative thinking. Evaluating decreases in depression through the lens of an emotion-focused practitioner is different given its emphasis on the human emotional experience; identifying, accepting, and changing "emotion schemes" are part of the core concept of emotion-focused therapy (Greenberg 2015), and progress is generally thought to be successful when patients develop increased awareness of their emotional experience and can distinguish between helpful and unhelpful emotions. These examples emphasize that the orientation in which you work is a key element of how you define—and thus measure—depression in these instances.

The following two mock clinical mission statements compare CBT and emotion-focused practices, respectively, to illustrate how depression may be operationalized within the context of each.

Cognitive-Behavioral Therapy

I specialize in the treatment of depression by helping patients understand how problematic thinking can impact their mood. When harmful core beliefs are addressed and changed, symptoms of depression, such as feelings of worthlessness, hopelessness, or irritability, begin to decrease.

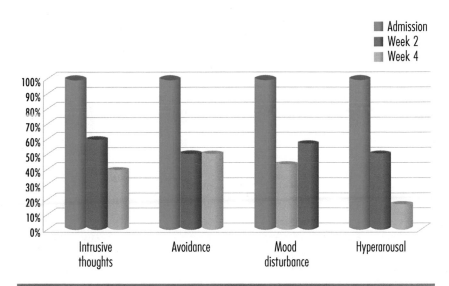

PLATE 1. *(Figure 3–3)* Bar graph example illustrating subscales showing the percent of posttraumatic stress symptoms reported.

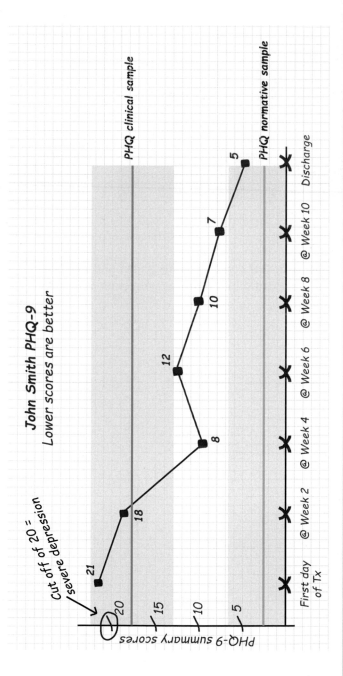

PLATE 2. *(Figure 4–4)* Visual inspection of therapeutic progress using standardized scores for reference.

PHQ-9=Patient Health Questionnaire–9; Tx=treatment.

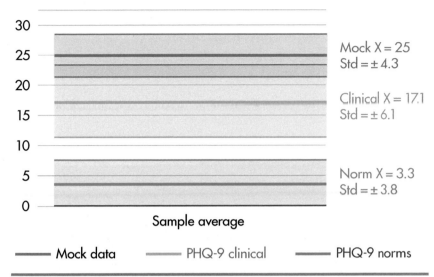

PLATE 3. *(Figure 5–1)* Demonstration of use measurement error using standardized scores for reference.

PHQ-9=Patient Health Questionnaire–9.

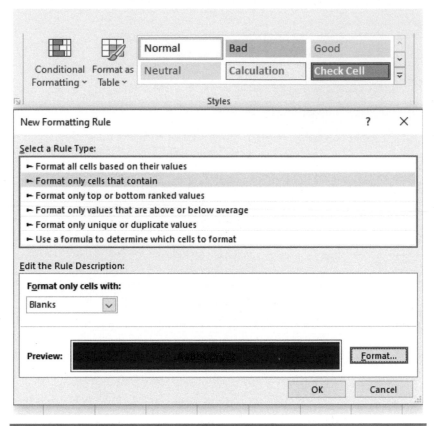

PLATE 4. *(Figure 8–3)* Microsoft Excel's point and click conditional formatting for identifying blank cells.

Emotion-Focused Therapy

I specialize in emotion-focused therapy for the treatment of depression. Patients become more aware of their emotions through our work together and learn to describe, regulate, and accept helpful versus unhelpful emotional states. Symptoms of depression, such as feelings of guilt, sadness, or fatigue, are reduced as the patients develop healthy ways of coping and reforming their personal scripts.

Identifying what you treat and how you treat it essentially lays the foundation for operationally defining your MBC program. This then guides your choice of the appropriate psychological tests for measuring your patients' progress. Because many psychiatric symptom scales are available to measure the same condition, deconstructing the mission statement into measurable component parts streamlines the selection of tests to best represent your practice and how you conceive psychotherapy. The more a chosen test aligns with your approach, the more meaningful your MBC program will be, because *you are the one responsible for interpreting therapeutic change.*

Appendix A presents a "Why-What-How Operationalization Worksheet" to help you deconstruct your clinical practice into measurable constructs. Table 3–1 is an example of how CBT therapists might complete the form to drill down to which psychotherapeutic change variables are important in their practice.

Operationalization is one of the harder tasks involved in implementing MBC. Detailing the specifics, conditions, and processes of practice requires a deep dig (with support from DSM or ICD) into how you identify distinctive features that make up the symptom condition. Combining both the symptoms of clinical presentation and your guiding practice orientation will add further dimension to how you would expect to observe change in these symptom presentations over time. Some conditions are more difficult to objectively define than others; for instance, one of the claims in the example mission statement refers to the treatment outcome of leading "well-adjusted, happy lives." If treatment goals comprise greater existential outcomes as part of the "why," then you'll want to add these into the measurable constructs. Phrases such as "reduced suffering," "successful recovery," or "happier life," are abstract and require careful consideration.

Operationally defining meaningful psychotherapy progress outcomes has been a constant in the field of psychology among theorists and diagnosticians alike. There is arguably more to meaningful psychiatric and psychotherapeutic progress than gauging treatment success as either the absence of disease or the reduction of psychiatric symptoms (World Health Organization 1946). A reduction in debilitating symptoms is indeed the driving force for patients to seek help, yet restoration of psychosocial and quality-of-life

TABLE 3–1.   Drilling down the clinical mission into measurable components

My why: professional mission statement

I believe that through the therapeutic process of identifying and challenging negative, harmful ways of thinking, patients can reduce their suffering and lead well-adjusted, happy lives. When harmful beliefs are addressed and changed, feelings of worthlessness, irritability, rejection, or worry begin to decrease while psychological states of confidence, self-esteem, and optimism become stronger.

What I treat: operationalizing conditions

Condition	Measurable constructs
Persistent depressive disorder	Apathy, hopelessness, pessimism, low motivation
Social anxiety	Avoidance, worrying about humiliation or embarrassment, subjective units of distress
Poor self-esteem	Low confidence, feeling inadequate, passivity
Well-adjusted life	Quality of life functioning, work fulfillment, stable relationships, healthy lifestyle

How I treat it: operationalizing approaches

Therapeutic method	Measurable constructs
Cognitive-behavioral therapy	Attitude, behavior frequency, insight, belief schema

functioning is also very important (Lam and Kennedy 2015). Functional mental health is greater than the sum of its presenting symptoms; it includes satisfaction with both interpersonal and social relationships and achieving a sense of identity, worthiness, and self-acceptance (Lambert 2010; Strupp 1963; Strupp and Hadley 1977; World Health Organization 1946).

Lam and Kennedy (2015) suggested that psychiatric treatment objectives are not met by obtaining simple symptom relief but through improved reported psychosocial functioning and quality of life. Numerous articles explore such topics, and some include validated scales that purport to measure such experiences. For an excellent read on the topic of operationalizing "recovery," consider McLellan's (2021) commentary on "Seizing the Moment to Improve Addiction Treatment" or Ashford et al.'s (2019) "Defining and Operationalizing the Phenomena of Recovery"; further discourse on operationally defining depression recovery is reviewed in Greer et al.'s (2010) "Defining and Measuring Functional Recovery From Depression."

The academic exercise to deconstruct your "why" is a worthy endeavor because it clearly transforms your vision into measurable component parts. It defines your treatment goals, outlines the expected milestones of therapeutic progress, and specifies the process by which change should take place. The art of operationalization is to take the qualitative, subjective, and, at times, ethereal nature of psychotherapy and put it through the objective, quantitative realm of substantiation.

Choosing Measures to Match Your Mission

Operationalizing your practice not only identifies specific elements of the psychological symptoms distinctive to your orientation and overall therapeutic approach but also serves to guide your measurement selection, rather than letting the test dictate your MBC program. There is a difference between simply grabbing the first depression scale you find (or choosing a depression scale because someone else told you to) and discovering the most appropriate depression scale specific to your clinical orientation through thoughtful consideration. Measures are nothing more than tools. Therefore, the tools you choose should align well with your overall practice so that the test data are simply natural extensions of the clinical interpretation.

Completing the Why-What-How Operationalization Worksheet helps you define the treatment conditions central to your clinical repertoire. For instance, which psychiatric condition(s) do you specialize in? Is it anxiety? Which subtype? Is it depression? Or do you view yourself more as a generalist? Outlining the psychiatric conditions in which you specialize establishes those objective "constructs," which can then be measured. Take specializing in clinical depression, for example: there are many available depression scales to choose from. Returning to the example in Table 3–1, after identifying the measurable constructs of depression, the clinician is equipped to explore depression scales that account for apathy, hopelessness, *and* low motivation. Subsequent review of depression measures, paying attention to items and subscales (i.e., variables), will aid in choosing the scale that best aligns with the clinical orientation and psychiatric criteria. Aligning clinical orientation with the MBC scale will provide meaningful interpretation of the patient's treatment trajectory.

Arguably, you may never find that one comprehensive measure to account for everything important to assessing a condition. However, conducting a thoughtful and thorough search, armed with a pragmatic approach to guide you, will yield a degree of confidence about choosing the most appropriate scales integral to your practice. Part III offers a compendium of accepted measures for psychiatric conditions and quality of life, along with open-source resources so that you may explore other options as well.

Know Your Audience for Effective Reporting

Psychometric data alone mean little unless they are used. The very premise of MBC is the edict to use patient self-report data in the context of treatment planning, progress management, and therapeutic outcomes. MBC is a new tool in our trade and, if used correctly, helps us do our jobs with greater ease, efficiency, and *clinical meaning*. Yet a finished product must have some purposeful application and set of instructions for its use. With that in mind, with whom do you plan to share the product of MBC? In other words, who is your audience? Who are the stakeholders in your practice who will 1) need to know, 2) benefit from, and 3) support your programming based on MBC output?

Identifying Stakeholders

Obviously, our patients are (or should be) the most important stakeholders in our practice. They stand to gain the most from their own personal MBC progress information and especially the complete MBC "report card," if you will. The next most important stakeholder is you, the treating practitioner. One of the indirect benefits of MBC discussed in Part I is the value-added opportunity to increase the therapeutic alliance between practitioner and patient (Dowrick et al. 2009; Fortney et al. 2015). Progress and outcomes data serve as a report card not only for your patient but also for you. Data captured through objective measures can also augment a working clinical hypothesis to enhance your patient understanding. Data are your friends.

Depending on your practice, other stakeholders will vary. Whether you are in private practice, a group practice, or a larger organization, the third most important stakeholder is often the one who holds the purse. This might be you, your board, or managed care. If there was any other reason to implement MBC besides its clinical utility, the ability to report outcomes with objective data certainly comes in handy when demonstrating the effectiveness of therapeutic programming to those with paycheck or reimbursement power. For example, for accredited practices, institutions such as the Commission on Accreditation of Rehabilitation Facilities (CARF) or The Joint Commission (TJC) will expect to review your MBC process. Having an established MBC program already in place when applying for accreditation will be an added bonus in your application, especially if you can aggregate patient data to demonstrate treatment fidelity. Clinical partners, families, schools, supervisors and supervisees, and even community partners may all represent stakeholders in your practice. Figure 3–1 (a blank version is available in Appendix B) is an example of a helpful and creative way to identify and list those who might be stakeholders in your practice.

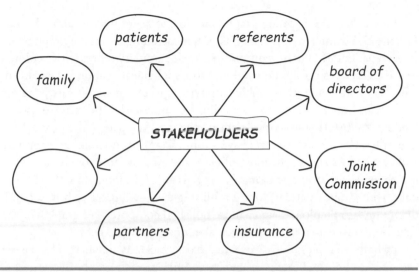

FIGURE 3–1.   Who are your stakeholders?

Tailored Stakeholder Reporting

You have collected patient data and scored it. Now what? What you do next is the art form of telling the story that MBC data provide. Do you write out an eloquent, qualitative report? Simply illustrate summary scores on a line graph? Talk about patient self-report data without visuals? The choice here is truly yours. How and with whom you share patients' MBC information will guide the method of presentation necessary to "reach" them. You don't want to spend all this time implementing MBC only to discuss the findings with a deer-in-headlights audience. Trust us on this: know your audience.

Visuals

By far, the easiest of all methods to convey patient data is through graphs and tables. When clearly denoted, graphs in particular are the output of choice for communicating progress, especially to the patients themselves. Most humans have gone through some form of educational system, which means they know (but have not always loved) report cards. When MBC data are plotted on a line graph, starting with pre-treatment status, they are easy to follow and understand change over time. As data points are added, patients come to expect and even look forward to seeing their progress. It is important at the outset, however, to take the time to explain what the scores on the graphs mean. Discussing the sub-scores and summary scores should suffice when reviewing patient progress; however, discussing the individual items of a scale sometimes may serve an important function, especially when clinically relevant (i.e., change in a test question on suicidal ideation).

Producing and updating graphs should not be an insurmountable task. For the DIY clinician, this can be as simple as adding a sheet of graph paper to each patient file and literally plotting their summary scores with a colored pen after each testing administration. More sophisticated approaches can entail a DIY data-generated graphic output using a computer software program (e.g., Microsoft Excel). If you are using a commercial MBC service, downloading and printing individual data graphs are often part of the product deliverables. Regardless, reported symptom changes over time are captured, and graphed visuals are the most efficient and effective tool for communicating therapeutic progress. Using Patient Health Questionnaire–9 (PHQ-9) data from a mock patient, John Smith, Figure 3–2 illustrates how a hand-drawn line graph plot (A) and a more polished computerized graph from an Excel spreadsheet (B) can effectively demonstrate MBC data.

In both examples, the x-axis and y-axis are clearly detailed. The clearer the denotation, the better the understanding. In each graph, the nature of the score is clearly indicated on the y-axis (i.e., PHQ-9 "summary" scores), the time intervals during which the self-report data were captured are listed on the x-axis, and a note that lower PHQ-9 scores means less depressive symptomatology is included in the title. It is always helpful to add extra information regarding cutoff scores to further gauge the extent and direction of progress. The severity cutoff score per the PHQ-9 is clearly demarcated so that both patient and therapist can glean the extent of progress and how the patient's reported depression compares with a clinical sample.

Choosing visuals to track symptom change is an elegant solution and can be easily explained to almost anyone. Line graphs are the preferred and recommended type of graph to plot *change over time*. Bar graphs, by comparison, although meaningful in their own right, should be used for categorical data or when comparing two or more groups (Dodge 2008), such as when categorizing patients by groups or clusters (e.g., demographic indicators) when reporting the overall effectiveness of a program (see Part IV). For individual patients, a bar graph may be applicable if you use an instrument with subscales or standardized scores. Figure 3–3 is a good example of how the reported domains of a PTSD measure, PTSD Checklist for DSM-5 (PCL-5), make better sense demonstrated by a bar graph than a line graph.

Each time a patient completes an MBC survey and the data are scored and plotted, reviewing the graphic data findings together augments the therapeutic process. Whether there is marked improvement, minimal improvement, or an increase in symptoms, discussing the clinical manifestations represented by the data is fodder for deeper clinical engagement. When thus integrated, MBC data give additional clinical meaning to the therapeutic process. For example, it is not uncommon to observe an increase in patients'

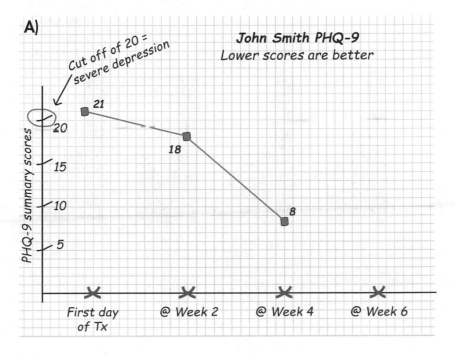

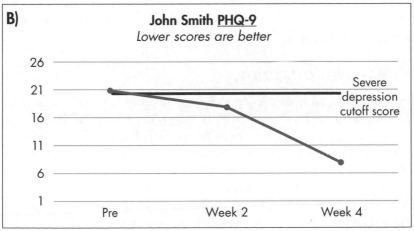

FIGURE 3–2. Plotting treatment (Tx) progress by hand (**A**) and captured and graphed using Microsoft Excel (**B**).

anxiety near the time of discharge. When queried, patients will speak about their fears of leaving the sanctuary of inpatient care; as a result, therapists often use this moment to review patients' progress, remind them of their enhanced coping skills, and validate their fears. Self-report data in this way can

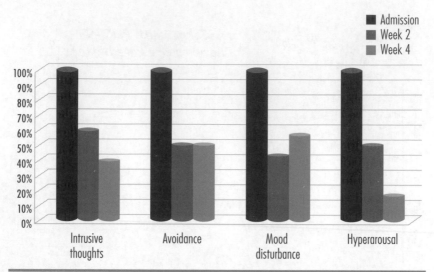

FIGURE 3–3.   **Bar graph example illustrating subscales showing the percent of posttraumatic stress symptoms reported.**
To view this figure in color, see Plate 1 in Color Gallery.

reveal what otherwise might not be openly shared during therapy. A visual uptick in anxiety captured on a graph can open up discussion and strengthen therapeutic alliance.

Qualitative Reporting

The qualitative psychometric report is fundamental to the assessment practice of most clinical psychologists. MBC is by no means a substitute for clinical psychological assessment, and likewise, there is little need to write the typical psychometric multipage narrative specific to patient MBC data. The need for a written report will most likely be dictated by the stakeholders who request it; thus, identifying their requirements will be key during MBC implementation. For the medical record, a therapeutic note incorporating MBC should require no more than an additional statement as to what was discussed while reviewing patient data progress (and, ideally, will include the graphs presented to the patient). For managed care reviews, copies of individual patients' graphed progress are usually sufficient. For accrediting institutions, CARF or TJC auditors will review the medical record looking for proof of MBC (i.e., graphs), any progress notes conveying discussions of the findings, and whether treatment plans were modified based on need. In most cases, a narrative report specific to each patient's MBC progress is unlikely to be requested, but that does not mean it will never happen. As

John Smith   **September 12, 2021**

Rationale
As standard procedure at Clinic XYZ, patients complete a series of assessments to augment the clinical process to further understand the clinical complaint, determine treatment course, and establish a baseline measurement of psychological status. Mr. Smith completed the assessment series on September 12, 2021, and the data were discussed with him on September 17, 2021, during a subsequent session.

Tests administered
Patient Health Questionnaire—9 (PHQ-9)
PTSD Checklist for DSM-5 (PCL-5)

Findings
PHQ-9
    The Patient Health Questionnaire—9 (PHQ-9) is a multiple-choice nine-item self-report scale used to determine the severity of depressive symptoms, using a 4-point Likert scale with responses ranging from "not at all" to "nearly every day." The higher the summarized score, the greater the reported depression severity. The PHQ-9 has strong validity and reported alpha coefficients ranging between 0.86 and 0.89.
    Mr. Smith's summary score of 21 is slightly above the cutoff of 20 for "severe depression." Patient tended to endorse items such as X, Y, and Z, and reported during feedback that these issues have been chronically affecting him for nearly 6 months.
PCL-5
    The PTSD Checklist for DSM-5 (PCL-5) is a 20-item self-report measure that assesses the 20 DSM-5 symptoms of PTSD. It comprises four subscale domains of re-experiencing, avoidance, negative mood, and hyperarousal. Validation studies confirm it has good internal consistency, from 0.56 to 0.77. A cutoff raw score is 39 for a provisional diagnosis of PTSD.
    In all four sub-categories, Mr. Smith endorsed significant distress with respect to intrusive thinking, avoidance of the issues, hyperarousal, and low mood associated with his trauma. The findings support a diagnosis of PTSD.

Summary and treatment plan
    The admission data resonate with Mr. Smith's expressed concerns during clinical interview; additionally, clinical observations also corroborate the data and his self-report. Due to his traumatic history, which likely remains unresolved, and despite Mr. Smith's efforts to manage stress with a variety of healthy coping strategies (i.e., exercise, journaling) in addition to maladaptive coping (i.e., isolation, progressively heavier use of alcohol), the unresolved trauma has likely manifested over time with increasing depression.
    During initial clinical interview, the patient and this writer have agreed to begin psychotherapy two times per week with the aim of understanding some of his deeper core beliefs that may be contributing to poor behavioral choices and thus interfering with his successfully "moving past" (his words) his trauma.
    Progress data capture will commence every 2 weeks or at the beginning of every fifth session (henceforth at 5 sessions, 10 sessions, 15 sessions, etc.) to track Mr. Smith's therapeutic gains.

FIGURE 3–4.   Sample qualitative report.

the practice of MBC expands, larger clinical programs, whether for-profit, nonprofit, or community mental health, may dictate their own policies regarding MBC reporting. We would be remiss if we did not offer a basic guideline for composing a qualitative description of patient data. The following is a list of general guidelines for composing a qualitative report, and Figure 3–4 illustrates how an initial report may be composed.

1. Rationale of the testing
2. List of the selected tests administered
3. Paragraph describing the test, including reported validity and reliability
4. Paragraph specific to patient's findings and what they mean
5. Summary and overall conceptualization
6. Action plan (how treatment may be tailored based on findings)

Summary

To get started with implementing MBC clearly requires forethought beyond simply administering a symptom scale to each client in your caseload. We can all collect data; it's what we *do with it* and how that matters. In the case of utilizing MBC as part of the clinical repertoire, these data offer vast potential to integrate what you do and how you do it with who you treat and whoever else needs to know. By operationalizing your orientation and approach, you solidify the foundation from which therapeutic growth occurs—which truly is the quantitative basis for each patient's story of progress under your care. The rest of getting started with MBC may be creative play for some or the drudgery of busy work for others: How do you illustrate patient progress, and how do you report those stories to other involved stakeholders?

Because you are the one responsible for interpreting therapeutic change, using the tools of MBC that align best with your practice gives you the *quantitative* advantage to the nuanced *qualitative* nature of psychotherapeutic care. The next step under your direction is ensuring that the methods by which you substantiate progress verifiably align with the treatment progress itself.

Chapter
04

Operations Infrastructure

AUGMENTING clinical practice to support a measurement-based care (MBC) program will likely be more of an iterative-reiterative process than a complete practice overhaul. To implement a meaningfully interpretable MBC program, the methodology by which therapeutic progress data are collected and the manner in which those data are used are important factors for successful practice. The time-series nature of MBC is essential if the data are to have meaning; thus, the methods to capture, review, and discuss patient data within prescribed timeframes provide the material from which the therapeutic story unfolds. Meaningful data collection requires a solid framework or infrastructure. MBC is no exception to this rule.

Basic Design Methodology for Clinical Practice

The structure to implement MBC ideally should fit into one's existing practice method, which typically comprises 1) a pre-treatment encounter, 2) the therapeutic intervention, and 3) a discharge process. These three conditions define the time-series in which MBC is implemented to assess for therapeutic change. This "pre-mid-post" practice method is akin to research methods utilized in evidenced-based practice (EBP) studies. One recognized within-subjects repeated measures design often utilized in EBP studies is the single-subject design (SSD), or A-B-A design. Because MBC is a data collection method that is integrated into psychotherapy, adapting the SSD approach to fit the framework of your practice may be the most elegant solution to launching MBC. Adjusting your intake process (or pre-treatment encounter) will require not only the addition of new MBC scales to obtain patient baseline status but also an update to your practice consent form.

Revisions to Consent

Before implementing MBC, it is necessary to revise your practice consent form to include a paragraph on MBC. The purpose of obtaining consent from psychotherapy patients is to make the terms of treatment clear and to outline any potential risks; the practice of MBC also falls within these guidelines. MBC is an assessment process achieved through data collection, and modifications to the consent should include considerations similar to those outlined in the informed consent of psychological assessment and behavioral research.

As discussed in Part I, MBC is an integration of the scientific method to inform and engage patients through measures and to substantiate the therapeutic process through the data acquired from those measures. Therefore, the risks and benefits that accompany some of the factors in psychological assessment and behavioral research must be disclosed during the informed consent process. A paragraph about MBC should include a brief statement that you practice measurement-based care as part of your psychotherapeutic approach and your justification for why this practice is beneficial. It is advisable to indicate which symptom scales you will use and how long it will take to complete them. Patients should be told that they will be expected to complete these measures in a routinized fashion that should also be explained (e.g., at the beginning of each session, through a patient portal every 2 weeks). It is important to add that their MBC data will be discussed with them as part of the therapeutic encounter to ensure that their course of treatment sustains therapeutic growth. There are few risks involved in completing symptom scales; however, the consent should include that people sometimes feel increased anxiety while responding to questions, as well as embarrassment, confusion, or frustration. Indicating that emotional responses to symptom scales are common but can be processed in the course of subsequent therapeutic encounters should assuage any uncertainty.

The paragraph explaining MBC should close with how patient data will be managed. Outlining steps for privacy protection, how data are stored, and steps taken to manage data after patient discharge are essential features in the consent. If your practice mission includes aggregating MBC data for quality assurance purposes, it is best to inform patients of this intention; often, a separate consent (or an embedded consent paragraph specific to obtaining permission to aggregate their deidentified information) for this purpose is appropriate. Finally, informed consent is both a legal and ethical agreement to promote patient-centered care and respect the autonomy and rights of patients to participate in treatment. Therefore, patients should be offered the option to *not* participate in MBC. If they choose to decline that part of the therapeutic process with you, it is important to note in the consent form that their decision will in no way affect the quality of their treatment.

Single-Subject Study Designs

The methodology of EBP research mimics real-world clinical practice methods. The SSD, as noted by Byiers et al. (2012), makes it ideal for clinical application. EBP studies embody experimental manipulation and control, much like large group studies, but the single-subject method (or "small-N" studies) focuses on studying individual responses in a small number of people. This means capturing nuances of change or response data that are often lost in the quantitative averaging of big-group research. Furthermore, and integral to the discussion when analyzing aggregated MBC, is that in SSD, *patients serve as their own statistical control.* SSD, on the surface, may appear similar to case study design; both are geared toward intensive focus on individual behavior. However, they differ with respect to method and analysis. The case study is qualitative in nature, often involving an intensive investigative analysis of an individual within a natural setting (Hamel 1993; Yin 2003). SSD, on the other hand, also intensively investigates an individual over time, but within the context of a controlled process while incorporating the use of assessments at prescribed times to determine change. Thus, the SSD structure lends itself beautifully to meaningful MBC.

The SSD method incorporates two important methodological features synergistic to clinical practice: 1) its prospective design and 2) the use of repeated measures. Collecting MBC data at pre-treatment or prospectively is essential; it not only serves as a baseline or starting point from which to compare patient progress but also is as close to a scientific "control" as we can get in the naturalistic, single-subject approach. We cannot control for all of the variables associated with patients' life history prior to their working with us, but certainly we can use their intake status as the starting point from which our therapeutic impact shows their progress. Not ascertaining patient status prior to the treatment course renders MBC basically ineffectual for determining the true extent of therapeutic change and outcomes. Therefore, it is critical to capture every patient's pre-treatment status before the first therapeutic encounter and to note the date for each. If patients complete their pre-treatment forms in the waiting room prior to their first therapy session, then it is important to further distinguish the time the assessment took place from the time the therapy session began.

The second important feature of SSD is its "repeated measures" method. This means identifying the time intervals during which treatment progress is collected and maintaining that plan across patients. Some EBP manuals offer guidance about when to administer symptom scales and some do not. The determining factors are your preferences for implementation and what works for your practice. This is an open "gimme," so to speak, but once you decide on the time-series method (i.e., prior to each session, biweekly, monthly), it is prudent that you abide by your own plan. The key to keeping data collection from overspilling into an unstructured, overwhelming miasma is to establish this infrastructure before launching MBC. Because moving targets make it hard to tell a sensible, consistent story, having all patients complete their MBC process in the same way yields a clean, defensible system of data.

Aligning MBC methods to capture therapeutic progress based on the tried-and-true SSD method is an excellent start to building your framework. The good news is that your practice structure is already likely similar to some variations of the single-subject approach and only minor tweaking will likely be required to effectively implement MBC.

There are many iterations of the single-subject A-B-A design, and we focus on two of these: 1) the A-B-A design and 2) the A-B-A-C-A design. Each lettered indicator in these designs denotes a stop or start in treatment phases or "study interventions." For the purpose of implementing these design methods for MBC, we suggest considering how to loosely adopt these treatment phase indicators as the general structure for capturing your own MBC data. In the following discussion, we consider these two designs of the single-subject method and how they may translate into practice.

A-B-A Design

In the A-B-A design, also known as a withdrawal or reversal design, the first A refers to a baseline phase in which no treatment is given, and the B refers to the intervention phase. The second A, as it pertains to study design, involves removing the intervention (B) to evaluate participants again without intervention exposure, thus attempting to assess for causation (Byiers et al. 2012; Zettle 2020). This allows researchers interested in the effects of a given intervention to observe the extent to which a participant returns to baseline after its withdrawal, thereby substantiating the intervention effects (Chiang et al. 2015). This method is guided by the hypothesis that behavioral change is due to an intervention and that the removal of that intervention will result in a return to baseline (thus experimental control). This allows researchers some space to consider causation.

In the real world of psychotherapy, it would be horribly unethical to remove an intervention while the patient is still under our care in order to test

TABLE 4–1. **A-B-A single subject design as framework for MBC in short-term psychotherapy**

A-B-A design	Test dates	PHQ-9 scores
A—Baseline/Intake	January 15	21
B—Interventional period (MBC collected every 2 weeks)	January 29	18
	February 12	8
	February 26	12
	March 12	10
	March 26	7
A—Therapy termination	April 9	5

Note. MBC=measurement-based care; PHQ=Patient Health Questionnaire.

its efficacy. Our therapeutic aim is behavioral and emotional change, and *change* is a result of *learning*. Therefore, we expect that our intervention (B) will have permanent, long-lasting effects even after treatment is completed. A return to baseline functioning after a course of psychotherapy might indicate treatment failure, because our patients did not "learn." The good news is that we are not doing EBP research but are loosely borrowing the methodology of data time-point acquisition with the A-B-A design. Adopting the A-B-A framework may serve well in those practices that use EBP manualized programs; the second A—removal of the intervention—is better postulated as representing the *termination* of psychotherapy. When patients complete psychotherapy, their treatment is essentially "terminated"; therefore, administering assessment during this discharge phase or after discharge could represent this second A. Continuing with the mock patient from Chapter 3, John Smith, Table 4–1 illustrates how the A-B-A design might provide the framework for a 12-week cognitive-behavioral therapy (CBT) program.

Table 4–2 illustrates how the A-B-A method might be used in short-term acute or subacute psychiatric care. The A-B-A design is well suited to represent the intake assessment (A), followed by psychiatric stabilization (B) and then discharge (A).

A-B-A-C-A Design

As overindulgent as it may appear, the lettered indicators of these SSDs can add extensions of alternating processes to the point of looking like DNA strands. The A-B-A-C-A design serves as another methodology for those practices that might use a more eclectic approach or in which adjusting medication over time is integral to achieving the correct treatment dosage. With respect to treatment research, the A-B-A-C-A design extends the logic

TABLE 4–2.   A-B-A single subject design as framework for psychiatric acute care

A-B-A design	Test dates	PHQ-9 scores
A—Baseline/Intake	January 15	28
B—Interventional period	5-day intensive inpatient	—
A—Therapy termination	January 21	17

Note.   PHQ=Patient Health Questionnaire.

of withdrawal/reversal designs to include more phases and more conditions for comparison (Byiers et al. 2012). Treatment begins with the A-B-A design, which is followed by a C-A design when changes to intervention occur. The second A phase here overlaps as both the withdrawal condition for the A-B-A portion of the experiment and the baseline phase for the A-C-A portion (Byiers et al. 2012).

In many ways, the method of the A-B-A-C-A design represents real-world clinical practice when the effects of an intended therapeutic approach do not result in symptom reduction as initially hoped, warranting a change to the treatment plan by introducing a different approach. Using the A-B-A-C-A method, the intervention can be modified or another intervention selected, and the effects of the new intervention can be measured. The Sequenced Treatment Alternatives to Relieve Depression (STAR*D) study relied on an extended form of the A-B-A-C-A design that allowed for a four-step protocol in which participants could switch therapy or augment their current treatment (Gaynes et al. 2008). The flexible single-subject approach of the STAR*D was designed to mirror real-world psychiatric and medical care and thus generalize findings accordingly.

In the research world, one is restricted from reporting causation using the A-B-A-C-A design because any relative or cumulative effects of each subsequent intervention cannot be scientifically controlled. The only conclusions that can be drawn are that one, both, or neither intervention was effective relative to baseline (Zettle 2020). MBC is not research, however, so we are not restricted in the same way. The A-B-A-C-A method for MBC structures the assessment time intervals for gauging when an alternate therapeutic approach may be introduced during the treatment trajectory. For example, should a patient report increased symptoms during one of the testing administrations in such a way as to cause the provider to change therapeutic course, that data point would become the second A, representing both termination of the current treatment approach and baseline status for the revised treatment approach. Table 4–3 illustrates how the A-B-A-C-A design

TABLE 4–3. **A-B-A-C-A single subject design as framework for MBC in psychotherapy**

Phases of therapy	A-B-A-C-A design	Test dates	PHQ-9 scores
Pre-treatment	A—Baseline/Intake	January 15	21
Treatment 1 progress	B—Interventional period	January 29	18
		February 12	8
Switch treatment approach	A—Withdraw intervention Establish baseline for C intervention	February 26	12
Treatment 2 progress	C—Interventional period	March 12	10
		March 26	7
Discharge	A—Therapy termination	April 9	5

Note. MBC=measurement-based care; PHQ=Patient Health Questionnaire.

accounts for this type of scenario. The flexibility afforded in this method in an MBC program adds clarity and dimension to interpreting progress data.

Single-Subject Study Interpretation

Basing your MBC data collection methods on the SSD method will ensure consistency and time sensitivity for capturing progress data. The approaches by which single-subject researchers tend to analyze and interpret data also provide useful guidelines appropriate for clinical application.

Visual Data Inspection

Analysis of data in SSD studies is often based on visual inspection. Simply comparing data points between two or more conditions does not really require parametric statistics (Paronson and Baer 1992). If you employ a data plotting process as illustrated by the line graphs in Chapter 3, simply sharing therapeutic progress with your patient is a good start to effectively employing MBC. However, Type I errors (i.e., failing to reject the null hypothesis or, in our case, assuming true change has occurred when it has not) are slippery fellows, and one should use caution when interpreting or signifying "change."

Three parameters should be employed when visually inspecting data: 1) the extent of change between data points (i.e., How big?); 2) the direction of that change or how progress is "trending" (e.g., Is my patient getting better or worse?), and 3) latency, such as identifying how long it took to observe a change in scores (Chiang et al. 2015). Each of these parameters can be discussed with your patient and used therapeutically to explore that patient's responses. Extending the therapeutic progress as outlined previously (see Figure 3–2A) for John Smith, we illustrate in Figure 4–1 how these three parameters of visual inspection can be addressed.

Visual inspection of John's data allows us to discuss the three parameters within the context of psychotherapy. For example, a small shift in John's self-reported depression symptoms is seen by Week 2, but by Week 4 the drop in reported depression is dramatic. Here we have identified 1) the extent of change (from a little bit to a big shift), 2) the direction of that change (i.e., reduction in reported symptoms), and 3) the time point in therapy when notable changes occurred (in this case, within 1 month's time). This plotting method is also useful when patients report an increase in symptoms. In John's example, there is an uptick in depressive symptoms halfway through his second month. The three parameters guide us to discuss the degree of worsening (both extent and trend), and this allows the therapist and patient together to explore what was happening during this time period when John likely took a "step backward" (i.e., latency). When instances such as these occur, it is important to review the MBC checklist in your medical record notation or treatment notes.

1. Did you identify and discuss the increase in symptom reporting?
2. Did you address changes to the treatment plan?
3. Did you note in the medical record which treatment modifications were made?

Using Metrics to Substantiate Treatment Progress

As discussed, reporting therapeutic progress to stakeholders is par for the course for today's mental health clinician. Indications of treatment gains (or losses) can be reported based on qualitative feedback, as indicated by visual inspection of MBC data. Measurement-based feedback can also be augmented by units of measurement, further substantiating therapeutic progress empirically. Using metrics to gauge progress is nothing new for treating physicians in their efforts to manage clinical interventions, especially with medication management (Chawla et al. 2001), physiological changes (Jaeschke et al. 1989), or disease-specific functioning (Wyrwich and Wolinsky 2000). At present, there are a few quantitative approaches one can employ to substantiate treatment progress using either simple calculations of change or a tiered approach to substantiating change.

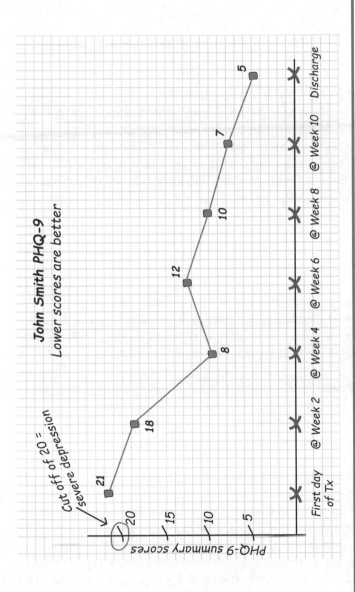

FIGURE 4–1. Visual inspection of therapeutic progress.

PHQ-9=Patient Health Questionnaire–9; Tx=treatment.

Simple Change Metrics

The appeal of SSD for the clinical practice is its elegant solution to collecting, plotting, visually inspecting, and discussing data. At the individual clinical practice level, conducting formal statistical analyses is not necessary. Nevertheless, for those who wish to employ quantitative methods to substantiate therapeutic change, a few hand-calculated metrics can be applied to the data. Two change metrics outlined here are percent change and reliable change index (RCI).

Percent change.   Calculating percent change between two data points is an excellent adjunct to augment the degree of therapeutic change. Percent change provides a percentage for the amount of change that has taken place (e.g., "Your depression score went down by 23%!"). How one calculates percent change is simple math: subtract the most recent score from an earlier score and divide its difference by the earlier score. This method can provide the degree to which one has reported a reduction (or increase) in symptoms over time. See Figure 4–2 for the formula.

The percent change metric can be incorporated as a parameter to gauge therapeutic milestones, as was used as one of the classifications structures for therapeutic progress in the STAR*D study. Basing progress as measured against baseline scores using the Hamilton Rating Scale for Depression and the Quick Inventory of Depressive Symptomatology (Self-Report) (see Table 7–8 for more information on these scales), modest improvements were classified by at least a 20% reduction in reported symptoms (Rush 2007), whereas positive treatment response was noted as a 50% reduction (Gaynes et al. 2008).

A word of caution is warranted, however, when interpreting percent change scores as "real change." The nature of the data collected from psychological tests is different from that of percent change calculations reflective of palpable change, for example, in education (e.g., "Look Ma! My grade improved 35%!") or income (e.g., "I'm making 13% more money this year than last"). Because symptom self-report data are more often ordinal, and neither ratio nor interval (like money), making claims to "real change" must be done with caution. When ordinal data are analyzed in larger studies, they are usually adjusted to account for a number of risks, such as measurement error, human variability factors, or other influences on test response. These precautions are put into place to avoid committing either Type I or Type II errors (seeing change where there is none and seeing no change where there is some, respectively).

Keeping the same conservative attitude when discussing the percent change of patient progress, we must avoid making sweeping claims of change

Percent change

$$\text{Percent change} = \frac{\text{New value} - \text{Old value}}{\text{Old value}} \times 100\%$$

If the result is positive, it is an increase.
If the result is negative, it is a decrease.

FIGURE 4–2.   Percent change formula.

TABLE 4–4.   **Sample of tracking percent change in Patient Health Questionnaire–9 (PHQ-9) scores over time**

Treatment phase	Date	PHQ-9 score	Change from pre-treatment, %	Change from previous sessions, %	Reviewed with patient?
Pre-treatment	January 15	21	—	—	√
2 weeks	January 29	18	–14	–14	√
4 weeks	February 12	8	–62	–56	√
6 weeks	February 26	12	–43	50	√
8 weeks	March 12	10	–52	–17	√
10 weeks	March 26	7	–67	–30	√
Discharge	April 9	5	–76	–29	√

but use this metric to show movement or approximations of change in therapeutic progress monitoring. The percent change statistic is an elegant indicator to substantiate progress and thus stimulate meaningful conversations.

Table 4–4 illustrates how one might track patient scores and progress over time using John Smith's Patient Health Questionnaire–9 (PHQ-9) data from Table 4–1. Two approaches to percent change are shown. The "Change From Pre-treatment" row uses the initial intake PHQ-9 score of 21 to gauge against each session progress. The "Change From Previous Sessions" shows percent change as it occurs twice weekly, to gauge the continuity of progress over time.

Reliable change index.   The RCI is the Cinderella metric to the stepsisters of the parametric statistical world; it is a hidden gem that is not widely considered. Those who know of it use it to assess *clinically* significant change in individual progress, as well as grouped data. Not only does the RCI pro-

$$RCI = \frac{X_{post} - X_{pre}}{\sqrt{2(S_{pre}\sqrt{1 - R_{xx}})^2}}$$

FIGURE 4–3.   **Reliable change index formula.**

vide a reliable indicator of whether change scores are due (or not) to chance, it also provides an iterative process for determining whether clinical significance has been achieved. The RCI takes the simple percent change calculation to new heights of gravitas.

Neal Jacobson and colleagues introduced the RCI in 1984 to encourage psychological science to consider the importance of clinical over statistical significance (Jacobson et al. 1984). When grouped data are analyzed for the purpose of generalizing outcomes to a population, the very process of employing parametric statistics comes with a price for understanding how a treatment under study has idiographic impact. The RCI, when used in studies with a large sample size, reduces threats to external validity by using the actual sample data against population test validity statistics to yield a metric that plots on the confidence interval of statistical probability (Jacobson et al. 1984). By incorporating measurement error into the calculation, the clinical significance of treatment progress can be taken into consideration. When applied at the individual clinical level, the RCI metric determines how much your patient's reported status has changed and whether that change is reliable and clinically significant (Zahra and Hedge 2010). The RCI dovetails beautifully within the parameters set forth by the SSD and, thus, MBC.

The RCI is a z-score metric based on the reported reliability of a test. It indicates whether and the extent to which change in scores assessed over time is due to therapeutic change or test measurement error (Evans et al. 1998). To calculate the RCI, you need two scores chosen from two assessment time periods and two statistics of the symptom rating scale used (these statistics should be included in the psychometric validation publication of your chosen test). These two statistics are 1) the standard deviation of the clinical sample used to validate the test and 2) the reliability coefficient of internal consistency, or Cronbach's α. See Figure 4–3 for the formula, where S_{pre} is the standard deviation of the test sample and R_{xx} is the reliability coefficient of the test.

The RCI is interpreted by observing whether the z-score falls above the 95% confidence interval of ±1.96, indicating that the change in scores may be due to therapeutic progress, or below ±1.96, indicating that the change in scores is more likely due to chance variation. Table 4–5 illustrates how

TABLE 4–5. Tracking reliable change index (RCI) of Patient Health Questionnaire–9 (PHQ-9) scores over time

Treatment phase	Date	PHQ-9 score	Change from pre-treatment score, %	RCI from pre-treatment score	Score ±1.96?
Pre-treatment	January 15	21	—	—	—
2 weeks	January 29	18	–14	1.05	No
4 weeks	February 12	8	–62	4.54	Yes
6 weeks	February 26	12	–43	3.14	Yes
8 weeks	March 12	10	–52	3.84	Yes
10 weeks	March 26	7	–67	4.89	Yes
Discharge	April 9	5	–76	5.60	Yes
Determining the denominator of RCI formula for calculation	$\sqrt{2(6.1\sqrt{1-0.89)^2}} = \underline{2.86115}$			Calculate the RCI by dividing the difference between two scores and dividing by 2.86	

one might incorporate RCI as part of MBC, based on our mock patient, John Smith. Both columns illustrating RCI and percent change in the table are based on comparing each subsequent score against the pre-treatment score. The clinical normative data published on the PHQ-9 (Kroenke et al. 2001) is used to demonstrate how to calculate RCI.

Tiered Approaches to Substantiate Change

Few researchers can be credited for innovative statistical approaches to assess psychotherapeutic progress at the individual level. Not too far back in the distant past, thought leaders like Neal Jacobson and Michael Lambert wrestled with the notion of how to substantiate therapeutic gains and losses using quantitative procedures to determine clinically meaningful changes in psychotherapy. The latter, in his quest to predict and thus prevent psychotherapeutic treatment failure, conceivably initiated the MBC movement.

The signal alarm. Concerned with the extent to which psychotherapy has negative rather than positive impacts for patients, Lambert launched a research agenda to study correlates of treatment failure. A by-product of this effort was the development and subsequent validation of the Outcome Questionnaire (OQ), a brief measure of psychological functioning delivered to practitioners in real time to gauge patient therapeutic progress. The OQ is based on the premise that treatment progress should be a measure of psychosocial functioning and not of symptom reduction alone. Extensive field testing ultimately resulted in a valid instrument for predicting treatment failure before it occurs by evaluating responses on a three-factor structure of 1) symptom distress, 2) interpersonal relationships, and 3) social role functioning (Beckstead et al. 2003; Hannan et al. 2005; Harmon et al. 2007; Hawkins et al. 2004; Lambert et al. 2004, 2005; Shimokawa et al. 2010; Whipple et al. 2003). The OQ output produces a color-coded alert system to notify the clinician to take prescribed action to ensure treatment success. This "signal alarm system" is predicated on an intraindividual change classification of "improved," "stable," or "declined" (Wyrwich and Wolinsky 2000), further comprising four-tiered notification outputs: 1) white tier (patient functioning at adaptive levels, consider termination), 2) green tier (patient on target therapeutically, continue treatment), 3) yellow tier (rate of therapeutic change not adequate, consider treatment adjustment), and 4) red tier (patient not making progress and at risk for dropout).

Clinical significance.   When using symptom scales other than the OQ, can similar tiered strategies be used to determine whether meaningful clinical change has occurred? Generally speaking, the answer is "yes," as long as both clinical and population normative data are provided for the chosen psychological test. In those instances in which norms are not available, strategies can be applied but must be interpreted with caution (Jacobson and Truax 1991). Combining the calculations of the RCI along with the normative data of a valid scale, Jacobson and Truax (1991) stipulated that clinically meaningful significance can be determined using a two-tiered approach for psychotherapeutic "recovery" by following two criteria: 1) the score difference between two time points must exceed the RCI (thereby inferring with 95% confidence that some amount of therapeutic change had occurred to reflect true change), and 2) the most current measurement score must fall within a range of normative values (Ferguson et al. 2002).

Others have used this method to develop guidelines for detecting change using the PHQ-9 (Belk et al. 2016; Jones et al. 2019), the Generalized Anxiety Disorder–7 (Belk et al. 2016; Bischoff et al. 2020), and the Short Form–36 (Ferguson et al. 2002). Referring back to Table 4–5, we can assess the likelihood of clinically meaningful change when incorporating normative values in John Smith's change metrics. Either a table or a graph can illustrate symptom change incorporating both clinical and normative data to substantiate patient progress. Figure 4–4 is an example. The shaded regions represent the range of values that vary around each clinical norm ($X=17.1, s=6.1$) and population norm ($X=3.3, s=3.8$) for the PHQ-9 (Kroenke et al. 2001).

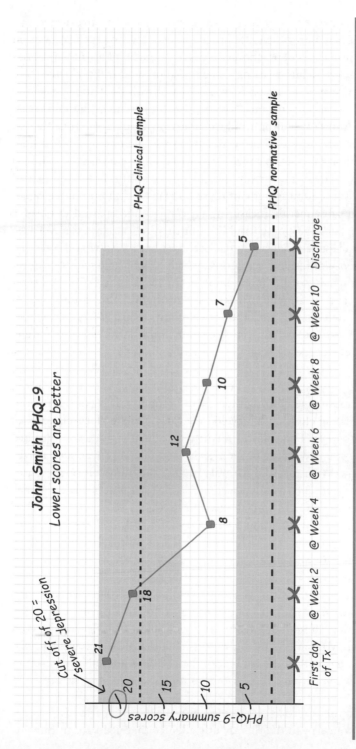

FIGURE 4–4. Visual inspection of therapeutic progress using standardized scores for reference.

PHQ-9=Patient Health Questionnaire–9; Tx=treatment.

To view this figure in color, see Plate 2 in Color Gallery.

Sustainable change. Tracking a score that meets the two-tiered approach criteria may not sufficiently proclaim recovery, however. A function of the healing properties of psychotherapy is the element of learning (i.e., behavioral change) to achieve lasting transformation, and in psychiatric care successful treatment is often considered achieved with the patient reaching remission and a return to "normal," or adaptive, functioning. Therefore, sustainability measured over time would further substantiate whether mental health gains are the result of successful treatment. The two-tiered system when using symptom scales to gauge recovery could be enriched by adding a third condition to determine psychotherapeutic recovery. This would entail taking the most recent measurement score that falls within normative values (criteria 2) and subsequently measuring it over a defined period to observe stability in reporting. Not only would this further indicate that some degree of sustainable adaptive functioning has occurred but it also would track the return or presence of residual symptoms, which is associated with risk of relapse and poor quality-of-life functioning (Lam and Kennedy 2004). Treatment *response* and treatment *remission* are distinguishable milestones in terms of reaching clinically meaningful endpoints (Rush 2007).

In Figure 4–4, the visual inspection of John Smith's data indicates a trend that his reported depression scores at week 10 and discharge are on track to signify sustained progress. How this is defined, and how the RCI criteria are determined and implemented overall, are opportunities for each clinical practice to establish when setting up its MBC program. It is not out of your reach as the treating clinician to develop your own practice formula to track therapeutic progress. The rules to identify therapeutic gradation outlined here can guide you in defining progress, whether it be improvement, inertia, or deterioration. With the RCI formula programmed into an open-source spreadsheet program such as Microsoft Excel, one can numerically track each patient's scores to compare with the patient's baseline score, an established clinical cutoff score, or with nonclinical normative values. Progress can be determined by the extent to which reported scores approach a "normal distribution" of functioning or clinical severity. Classifying scores as outlined by Lambert and Jacobson is only part of the MBC experience.

Although it may be riveting to some to get lost in the weeds of data and all the cool ways to use it, it is important not to lose the purpose of MBC, which is to utilize these methods in order to therapeutically engage your patients. When MBC alerts us to progress changes, it behooves us to discuss these findings within the context of the patient's mental health status. For example, when patients report inertial forces or potential failure:

- How might our approach to therapy improve for the patient?
- Are there concerns in the therapeutic alliance that need attention?

- Have outside events taken place that may have contributed to mental health decline?
- Have medication side effects interfered with quality of life?

Likewise, for success:

- What seems to have been working in therapy?
- In what ways have learned skills served the patient, and can these be applied to other areas of the patient's life?

With particular attention to treatment success, Jacobson and Truax (1991) urged caution when reporting recovery. In some cases, especially for patients with chronic mental health conditions, a "return to normal functioning" may not always be realistically achievable; accordingly, during therapeutic goal setting, one may wish to define success as reaching goals toward adaptive functioning or enhanced quality of life. Caution is warranted when using categorical markers to gauge clinically significant change. Although a far cry more informative than relying on statistically significant indicators (for the very reason that clinically meaningful individual change can never be extracted from statistically significant changes measured in aggregated samples), surmising meaningful change should still incorporate any individualized nuances presented by each unique patient. Creating an individual RCI calculus per patient will allow the use of individual patient scores ideographically to compare patients' own progress within the range of their own computed findings. The PHQ-9 data progress outlined in Table 4–5 is a good example of using the patient's own scores to determine the extent of measurable progress.

Application Approaches

By now, you should be well positioned to begin your MBC program. Understanding and appreciating the nuts and bolts of implementation, such as operationalizing your practice mission, choosing the appropriate MBC data collection methods, and using basic analysis, should help you determine your bandwidth for either setting up your own program or choosing a fee-based online platform that aligns with your business model. A firm knowledge of the step-by-step methodology to implement MBC, despite the size of the practice, will either prepare you to set up your own data collection methods or guide you in asking important questions for commercial data platforms. Either way, by now you are ahead of the proverbial curve.

To wrap up the "how" of MBC operations, we now consider which MBC protocol approach best suits your theoretical orientation, practice structure, and costs of doing business.

Configuring Your MBC Structure

Depending on the interdisciplinary nature of the group practice, defining the clinical vision, choosing measures, and presenting data may take on an added yet collective effort. Several MBC approaches can be implemented based on practice vision and need: 1) the customized individual protocol, which is to administer symptom rating scales specific to the presenting problem unique to each patient, 2) the collective standard protocol, which is to use a common measure to assess all your patients, irrespective of presenting problems, and 3) the comprehensive standard protocol, which is to use a battery of various measures to assess all your patients in a standard fashion. Obviously, the shorter the compilation, the less time it will take to administer and score, and vice versa.

Customized Individual Protocols

MBC can be simply woven into a clinical practice by choosing only symptom rating scales specifically for tracking patients' presenting conditions or a patient-centered customized approach to tracking their progress. In this method, one chooses only those symptom scales specific to each case presentation, such as using depression scales for patients seeking treatment of depression, or trauma symptom measures for those being treated for PTSD, or a combination of scales depending on the complaint.

One of the directives of patient-centered care is to tailor treatment specific to individual need. This form of personalized medicine spans from private practice to acute psychiatric stabilization. Therefore, the use of MBC from an individualized approach could be implemented to gauge symptom reduction specific to the goals of each patient. MBC in this instance uses symptom scales specific to each individual case, using a measurement formulation that starts and stops uniquely with each patient. Case open, case closed, with supportive quantifiable data substantiating treatment gains, progress, or losses *specific to tracking the identified symptom presentation* and verifying outcomes for communicating with managed care and patient alike.

Although simple, approaching MBC using this method also has its disadvantages. The upside is that this constitutes the more elegant solution, comprising in some cases just one or two scales to track therapeutic progress. The downside is twofold. First, use of single-symptom scales will likely fail to identify factors associated with comorbid mental illness. Second, any future plan to aggregate data to establish quality assurance, determine practice fidelity, or report overall programmatic effectiveness will be undermined by having a varied mixed bag of data.

With respect to clinical management and precision psychiatry, the need to anticipate psychiatric comorbidity in patient presentation is quickly becoming standard practice (Gamse 2019). Despite knowing the extent to which polygenic or environmental risk factors play a role in mental health issues, it is likely that up to 40% of patients will present with additional psychiatric conditions within the first year of diagnosis (Plana-Ripoll et al. 2019). What patients report during an intake assessment may not account for underlying issues for which they do not yet have insight or that you observe clinically. Limiting the implementation of symptom rating scales specific to primary treatment goals discussed at intake diminishes the opportunity to capture both nascent comorbid conditions and existing, yet underlying, issues. Of course, one could argue the logic of adding on symptom measures as treatment progresses and new symptoms present, but the cost is losing out on obtaining a multifaceted, "prospective" pre-treatment status and managing an expanding measurement-based process per patient. This approach can quickly become unwieldy; what starts out as an elegant approach can take on circuitous complications.

Not accounting for psychiatric comorbidity may be the most important downside to the customized individual protocol. Another downside may exist for those practices that want to expand their clinical operations. Neglecting to standardize measurement selection across all patients will negatively impact the collection of consistent data necessary for establishing program fidelity. For most private or small-group practices, the need to aggregate patient symptom data for reporting program fidelity may not be applicable; in these instances, MBC implementation at the individual, customized level may be the acceptable paradigm. For those practices in which reporting program fidelity is a practice objective, whether for analyzing quality assurance or demonstrating program effectiveness for accreditation, the "simple" MBC approach of administering one or two symptom scales specific to each patient condition will result in a complicated, time-consuming process to organize data and defend glaring data collection holes and will limit the ability to tell a consistent story about the practice's therapeutic value.

Collective Standard Protocols

One way to establish data consistency across all patients is to implement a collective standard approach to MBC. This method, like the customized individual protocol, requires little extra time and resources to establish. In fact, it may be a bit easier to implement the collective standard approach because it uses only one common measure to assess patients, irrespective of presenting problems, which saves time because there is no "picking or choosing" which measure for which patient.

Scales that fall under the "collective standard" are those multidomain, global, or multidimensional measures that purport to assess symptoms across a broad perspective. In Chapter 7, "Psychometrically Sound Scales," a list of these stand-alone measures is provided in Table 7–1, and various multidomain assessments are described in detail under the "Commercial Packages" sub-heading. The theoretical justification for developing many of these measures is based on recognizing psychiatric comorbidity and the multifaceted nature of effective psychotherapy. Assessing quality-of-life functioning, relational satisfaction, stress, and overall well-being in conjunction with psychiatric conditions promotes the balance of clinical and functional mental health (Jerrell 2005; Maruish 2013; Schmit and Balkin 2014). Self-report multidomain measures tend to be less diagnostic than specific symptom scales (few if any psychological tests are truly diagnostic), but the benefit to implementing a broader, all-encompassing measure is that it may capture subtle nuances in behavioral change in addition to addressing the shortcomings identified in an individualized approach with respect to psychiatric comorbidity.

Another benefit to using a collective standard approach is the ability to assess potential characterological or functional strengths that patients may not have recognized. It is not unusual for patients who are overwhelmed by emotional suffering to overfocus on their presenting problems without being aware of how their condition impacts other aspects of their lives. In many cases that we have observed directly, severely distressed individuals typically are surprised when shown their profiles from a multidimensional measure illustrating the presence of other adaptive (or maladaptive) functioning behaviors of which they were not aware. One of the fundamental assumptions of MBC is its function to promote deeper understanding or insight; the use of a global scale is likely to evince this sort of outcome.

What is lost in specificity is gained in the standardized general administration of the same scale across all patients. At the aggregate level, MBC data will provide consistently themed deliverables necessary to support quality assurance analysis, verify practice fidelity, and report overall programmatic effectiveness. Most global scales can be further analyzed by subscale, allowing for deeper consideration of which aspects of mental health or illness are affected by the treatment approach. Additionally, whether the practice is private, group, community, or institutional, those that endorse holistic, eclectic, or integrative approaches to psychotherapy can capitalize on multidimensional scale outcomes because the very nature of the assessment can substantiate the multifaceted approach to therapeutic healing.

The downside to the collective standard protocol is what is lost due to convenience. If the global multidomain measure superficially accounts for psychiatric concerns, measurement of the extent of symptom progress or status of remission is reduced. Rush (2007) warned that itemized symptoms scales are better than global scales with respect to tracking patient reported side effects of medication management as well as tracking reported symptom improvement due to psychotropic medications.

Comprehensive Standard Protocols

Approaches to MBC implementation can be further expanded by compiling a set of valid measures into a questionnaire battery. This approach typically mirrors epidemiological strategies to capture as much data as possible in order to dig deep in all sorts of ways to understand one's population of interest. At the psychotherapeutic level, a comprehensive approach would best apply to large, institutionalized programs, whether community-based, for-profit, or nonprofit, ranging from community outpatient programs to large national corporations overseeing many behavioral health care facilities. What drives the selection of a comprehensive standard approach is a thoroughly (operationally) defined practice mission and access to available resources.

To some extent, the comprehensive MBC protocol is an amalgamation of its two smaller counterparts. Rather than use a specific multidimensional self-assessment tool, the comprehensive approach obtains its multidimensional nature by compiling valid symptom scales to meet its MBC mission. This approach allows for both breadth and depth: breadth in terms of maintaining an integrative or comorbid perspective of mental health, and depth in terms of using reputable measures targeting specific psychiatric conditions. Others have suggested that a comprehensive approach to MBC addresses symptom side effect management, quality-of-life functioning, and mental health progress (Lam and Kennedy 2015; Valenstein et al. 2009; Zimmerman et al. 2012) to promote understanding, treatment planning, and therapeutic progress at the individual level while contributing to a clinical aggregated data bank to provide ample practice-based evidence for outcomes, program fidelity, and quality assurance at the program level.

Without the proper resources, the comprehensive standard approach is likely not readily obtainable. Reaching multiple users at multiple sites requires ingenuity with respect to automation, staffing, scheduling, and clinical onboarding. Big data are expensive to collect, manage, and analyze. Practical operational challenges aside, this approach signifies an MBC gold standard because of its scope in assessing multiple layers of mental health, psychosocial functioning, and health-related quality of life. From a global perspective, the behavioral health field could benefit exponentially from those larger mental health institutions that implement comprehensive MBC practices and report their outcomes through valid reputable analyses. Patient progress data coming from well-organized systems can propel the behavioral health field to legitimate new heights pertaining to best practices, enhancing managed care deportment, and informing the general public and politics alike about the veracity of mental health conditions, ultimately effectively challenging stigma.

Commercial Platforms

Choosing a commercial data analytics firm to collect, manage, and report patient data is rapidly becoming a necessary decision-making process in any clinical practice, no matter how large or small. Online data platforms have appeal in terms of time savings, ease of access, and administration, and most have qualified staff knowledgeable in psychological testing, methods, and data analyses. The downside to employing a fee-based program is, well, the fees. Fee structures can vary from price per-patient-per-stay, to price per-practitioner-per-month. In some instances, the fees are annual subscriptions that can reach into the thousands of dollars annually. As mentioned at the beginning of this chapter, MBC is fast becoming big business.

The MBC methods discussed in Part II are based on traditional behavioral health research and practice; there are no trade secrets or patents for data collection methodology, so aside from proprietary program coding, platform trademarks, or assessment copyrights, there is little that would justify the high cost of doing business with a commercial data analytics firm. Nevertheless, in many instances, fee-based online platforms may be the best solution for a clinical practice. Having read this book makes you an informed consumer. Ask the hard questions, demonstrate your MBC aptitude, and choose wisely. A few good questions to consider asking a commercial MBC data platform are:

1. How do you manage deidentified data? In what ways do you uphold HIPAA strategies to protect patient information?
2. Who owns my patient data? May I obtain the aggregated data at any time? Are there additional costs to downloading my patient data bank? What programs do you use to store data? Are these accessible to the end user?
3. What are your data security measures? How can you assure me you will protect my data from a data breach? How will you manage ransomware should your platform get hacked?
4. May I choose symptom scales or global measures not available in your inventory? Is there an extra cost for customizing my account?

Table 4–6 provides an alphabetical list of commercial data management businesses that advertise MBC solutions for mental health clinicians and practices. This list was compiled through a browser search using terms such as "MBC companies," "mental health data services," and "MBC analyses." None of these commercial websites is affiliated or has a relationship with either author.

TABLE 4–6. Commercial data management businesses specializing in measurement-based care

Company name	Website
Blueprint	www.blueprint-health.com
Code technology	www.codetechnology.com
Greenspace	www.greenspacehealth.com
Mindstrong	mindstrong.com
Mindyra	www.mindyra.com
Mirah	www.mirah.com
MyOutcomes	myoutcomes.com
NeuroFlow	www.neuroflow.com
Opeeka	www.opeeka.com
Owl Insights	www.owl.health
Sheppard Pratt	www.sheppardpratt.org
Total Brain	www.totalbrain.com
Tridiuum	tridiuum.com
Valant	www.valant.io
Vista Research Group	vista-research-group.com

Summary

Psychotherapy and psychiatry are genuine practices in which humans help other humans. There is an artform to this work that flows through a beginning, middle, and often "end" period in these relationships. This flow process is akin to how an added procedural layer such as MBC can seamlessly weave in. Regardless of the MBC protocol you choose, adopting standardized methodology to capture baseline functioning, intermittent progress, and treatment complete status are necessary requirements to accurately, reliably, and defensibly tell the story of therapeutic progress. MBC data, when captured systematically, seasons the fusion of clinical observation and patient progress insight with substantiated support for the extent of therapeutic gains, in what direction, and specifically when such changes took place. The data you collect does not have to be static if you choose it not to be. Using MBC findings in dynamic ways, such as through reliable change indicators augmented by clinical and normative data parameters, serves to guide you and your patient on their journey toward improved functioning.

Like any tool, its proper care with proper use can result in a meaningful construction—or in our case, meaningful outcomes.

PART III

The WHAT

The "Measures" in Measurement-Based Care

Chapter
05

Overview of Psychometrically Sound Measures

THERE are numerous texts, both old and new, that painstakingly delve into the world of psychometric testing. There are also tomes dedicated to the standardization practices of research methodology. Both categories are integral to measurement-based care (MBC) and deserve attention. Our promise to you, however, is to spare you the deeper minutiae of these academic disciplines; our aim is that you garner a general appreciation for what a "psychometrically sound" scale is and the methodological importance of test administration.

According to the Institute of Medicine (2015), *psychometrics* is the scientific study to develop, interpret, and evaluate psychological tests "to assess variability in behavior and link such variability to psychological phenomena" (p. 95). Psychometrics establish the qualities that make a test psychometrically sound, thus becoming a "good" test. In this chapter, we outline some of those features as a helpful guide for making MBC test selections.

Overview of Basic Psychometrics

There are several hurdles to jump when it comes to test construction, such as factor analysis, validity testing, determining reliability, and establishing norms, among others. The good news is that a wide breadth of symptom measures already exists, and some are very well-known and accepted, which means you do not have to develop your own. Nevertheless, in your quest to choose the right measures, you should become familiar with what makes a measure psychometrically sound. Neglecting to consider these factors in your MBC program can be the difference between gaining or losing respect and credibility with your colleagues or between landing or losing an insurance contract.

Validity

Test validity comes in many shapes and sizes. We focus here only on those facets of validity that are specifically important to guide you in choosing reputable symptom scales. Subcategories of validity, such as criterion, predictive, face, or discriminant, are not defined in this book. However, if your curiosity is piqued, it is best not to search the variations of validity without having a solid textbook on psychological testing on hand (a favorite is *Psychological Testing* by Anastasi and Urbina [1997]). The many internet blogs and opinions defining the variants of validity will only result in deeper confusion, disdain for psychometric test construction, and a headache.

Establishing the validity of psychometric tests accounts for the confidence and accuracy of what a measure *measures*. Arguably, the most important of all validities is *construct validity*, which is typically demonstrated when a particular test measures the condition, trait, or ability that it was intended to measure. "Construct" in this regard represents some underlying theme, symptom, or characteristic, as well as representing constructs such as satisfaction, attitude style, or quality of life. As William Trochim (2020) described, construct validity is "the approximate truth of the conclusion that your operationalization accurately reflects its construct." There's that *operationalization* word again. This is a good reminder of why taking the time to operationalize your clinical practice is important: operationalization is the basis of validity.

For a psychometric test to be valid, it must go through a rigorous process to collect theoretical information of a construct (or trait), analyze the consistency of study participant responses, and determine how well the test correlates with other measures known to assess the same construct (Anastasi and Urbina 1997). When reviewing the literature to determine whether a test you want to use is valid, authors will report the statistical findings they used to quantify construct validity. Most often, a correlation or "validity coefficient" will be reported to represent how strong the relationship is between two tests, especially if the target test was measured against another test that is already accepted as measuring the same construct. This latter effort signifies *concurrent validity testing*, which demonstrates how well one instrument compares with another that measures the same or similar constructs. The intersection of *construct* and *concurrent* validity is often what guides proper choice of valid measures. When selecting your test for MBC, review the literature for the validity coefficient; generally, a strong relationship will show a correlation of 0.8, a moderate relationship 0.6, and a weak relationship 0.4 (Rogers and Nicewander 1988).

Another statistic used to quantify construct validity is confirmatory factor analysis, especially for multiscaled measures. Confirmatory factor analysis is a process that yields how well the data from an assessment "fit" a specific theory-derived model. It was developed by Jöreskog in 1969 and has largely replaced the painstaking construct validity testing of Campbell and Fiske's 1959 Multitrait Multimethod Matrix (MTMM). If you read about the validity of a test and see MTMM referenced, don't be alarmed; it's just validity testing. The ways in which the strength of confirmatory factor analysis is reported can vary with statistics, such as chi-square, goodness of fit indices, comparative fit index, or root mean square error of approximation (Thompson 2004). Articles addressing validity testing using these methods will use significance level probability statistics (P values) to indicate the degree of fit.

Reliability

Test reliability is about consistency. For this book, understanding two aspects of reliability is important. First is the consistency of the actual test items, which is referred to as *internal consistency*. The internal consistency of a test is the extent to which all scale items measure different aspects of the same attribute; in other words, how interrelated are each of the test questions? The second aspect is the repeatability of the test, or the consistency of the test results obtained over time taken by the same test taker. This is also known as *test-retest reliability* (Anastasi and Urbina 1997).

Both aspects of reliability are important to MBC. If the assessment you use has established reliability, and your patient completes it at varying time points with differing results, then (voila!) a meaningful trend in therapeutic response warrants consideration. In other words, the change in the scores of a reliable test is not due to an error of the test (because it is *reliable*), so the change in scores must be due to something else (in this case, therapeutic progress).

Like validity, to establish test-retest reliability, the same group of participants must go through a rigorous methodological process of testing and retesting under the same conditions on differing occasions. When reviewing the literature to determine whether a test you want to use has repeatability, authors will report this type of reliability with a Pearson's correlation, the value of which ranges from 0.00 (no correlation) to 1.00 (perfect correlation). The higher the Pearson's correlation, the better the test-retest reliability. A test with good test-retest reliability will also correct for practice effects, which, as threats to internal validity, are influences on subsequent testing by virtue of repeated exposure to the test itself. Practice effects may be more of a nuisance for repeated performance measures rather than symptom measures, but they must be taken into consideration when reviewing the time-series nature of MBC.

Internal consistency reliability is reported as a Cronbach's α coefficient (Cronbach 1951). Similar to Pearson's coefficient, Cronbach's α also determines the strength of a test's inter-item consistency. Articles will report the α coefficient, ranging from 0 to 1, to report the overall measure's reliability. As a guideline, if the scale items are too independent from each other (i.e., they do not relate well to measure the given construct), then the α coefficient will be 0 or close to 0. If the items *do* relate well and capture a good representation of the construct, then the α coefficient will be close to 1.0. Generally, α coefficients <0.5 are considered unacceptable, whereas an α of ≥0.7 supports confidence in the test's internal consistency (Tavakol and Dennick 2011).

Normative Group Data

Becoming familiar with data norms when reviewing test selection is another important consideration. Worthwhile measures should not only demonstrate robust reliability and validity but also provide descriptive information concerning normative data (e.g., mean averages, standard error) about the populations in which the tests were evaluated. Many psychological tests and psychiatric symptom scales publish established normative data. These norms provide guidelines against which patients' scores are compared, thereby fostering interpretation. Without the population or clinical norms, how might one interpret, say, a summary score of 18? If a test you choose does not have established norms, then it is acceptable to use the study data from which the test was validated.

On Measurement Error and Interpretation

It is generally accepted that psychological tests are approximations of what they propose to measure, such as beliefs, attitudes, or moods. Unlike height, with its clearly accepted objective forms of measurement, there is no hard-and-fast rule to measure quality of life. In the world of psychometric testing, there is a theoretical notion that scores are composed of 1) true score and 2) error. The "true score" is a hypothetical representation of one's actual score *sans* testing error and random error (Institute of Medicine 2015). With

MBC, the interplay between testing error and true scores when employing ordinal response scales is important to consider (Fischer and Milfont 2011). Response options in symptom scales are most often Likert-type scales, and the range of anchor points typically varies from scale to scale. For example, if a patient's average summary score from a symptom scale is a 3, what does that 3 really mean when calculated on a 0–5 scale, 1–4 scale, or 1–10 scale? This can pose further problems when using more than one measure with differing answer options. Without knowing the normative data, whether population norms or clinical norms, interpretation would be rather difficult.

Taking measurement error into consideration when interpreting patient data can be a useful yardstick. We are all familiar with mean scores as factors that describe the central tendency of a group, but it is the standard error that allows for deeper interpretation. The standard error is about variation; it measures the extent to which a set of sample means disperse around a population average. The standard deviation works the same as the standard error, but on a smaller scale.

Allow us to create a fictitious account of aggregated depression scores to show how standard error helps with interpretation. After grouping a subset of patients' data together, it is easy to calculate a single metric to represent the average of their scores (i.e., group mean). The group's standard deviation is calculated by squaring the distance of each patient's score against the mean score, adding those up, and dividing that number by the sample size. In this fictitious sample, using Patient Health Questionnaire–9 (PHQ-9) data, the preadmission PHQ-9 average is 25 and the standard deviation is 4.3. Because the standard deviation shows how the scores vary (i.e., variance), that 4.3 means your patients' scores typically fall within ±4.3 points of the average of 25, thus ranging between 21.7 and 29.3.

Using this example, if you take your patient data and compare it with the normative data published on the PHQ-9 (Kroenke et al. 2001), you will be able to gauge the extent to which your patients' scores are unusually high, unusually low, or in the average range of the expected clinical or population norms. The clinical norms established in the PHQ-9 validity paper were those assessed in a sample of patients with diagnosable depression, and the reported mean was 17.1, with a standard error of 6.1. This means that for the 41 participants in this study who were clinically depressed and took the PHQ-9, scores typically ranged between 11 and 23.2. Why is this important? Because it tells you quite a bit about your patients:

1. Their PHQ-9 average of 25 is 8 points higher than the *expected mean* of the clinical sample, and their average is above the highest range variability of 23.2 in the clinical norm group. In fact, those in your practice who scored in the lowest range were comparable with the higher range in the

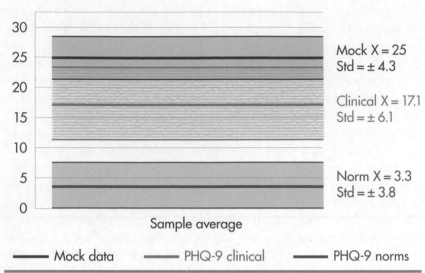

FIGURE 5–1. **Demonstration of use measurement error using standardized scores for reference.**

PHQ-9=Patient Health Questionnaire–9.
To view this figure in color, see Plate 3 in Color Gallery.

PHQ-9 study clinical sample. You can likely report that, based on the PHQ-9, you typically work with a severely depressed population. See Figure 5–1 for a visual illustration.

2. There is a modest 1.8-point difference between your group's standard deviation of 4.3 and the clinical standard error of 6.1. This could mean that you are working with a more homogeneous patient population than was expected in the PHQ-9 clinical population. It may also suggest that the PHQ-9 will be a reliable tool for you because the standard error of a measure is a function of test reliability.

3. Once you begin to collect progress data, at each point during the treatment trajectory you will be able to track just how much your patients are improving by comparing their scores with the PHQ-9 nonclinical normative scores. At some point, you might be able to use the nonclinical population norms from the PHQ-9 to gauge the extent to which your patients are approaching improvement. This approach demonstrates how to gauge treatment progress using a two-tiered approach, as described by Jacobson and Truax (1991).

Using published scores to interpret progress does not require amassing a collection of patient data; individual scores can be compared against the normative data. In fact, applying a test's normative data as part of your visual inspection aids well in interpretation. Referring back to Figure 4–4 in Part II, the simple line graph used to illustrate PHQ-9 progress also included both population and clinical variation spread to demonstrate the extent of progress as compared with clinical and normative ranges.

Parsimony

In the 14th century, William of Ockham suggested that simpler theories of logic (or explanation) that explained the entirety of a phenomenon were preferred over verbose entities *multiplied without necessity* (Epstein 1984). Many academic fields have since adapted the principle of parsimony, or "Ockham's razor," into their conventions, statistics, and psychology. For MBC, parsimonious measurements—those that best assess a condition with the fewest number of variables—should be a guiding principle when considering the right measures. As mentioned in Part I, Zimmerman and McGlinchey (2008) advised selecting scales that are brief and easy to complete. Therefore, during your hunt for the perfect scale, parsimony guides us to choose not just the briefest measure but the briefest measure with compelling test construction that best accounts for the condition of interest. Short and sweet is pleasantly brief and relevant.

Ease of Administration

The ease of assessment administration comprises two things: 1) the time and effort your patients need to complete the assessment and 2) the time and effort you need to proctor, score, and document the data. The easiest administration may be the one that ends up being the more expensive one if you decide to contract with an online commercial MBC company. Later in this section we outline several of these companies. For a busy psychotherapy clinic, hiring this sort of service may have its appeal because patients simply log in to a Web-based platform and complete the survey(s), and all you have to do is access the data output, which already has been scored, analyzed, and interpreted. Possible drawbacks to this option are not only cost but also loss of control over which measures you want to use, because many companies offer preset measures and charge more for customization.

The good news is that collecting patient self-report through traditional paper and pencil measures yields the same data output as the fancier automated programs. Therefore, choosing the method of administration is an important business decision. A do-it-yourself approach may save a lot of money, especially if you select an assessment in the public domain, but the cost will be your time or your staff's time to score and report or graph the results. The shorter the assessment, the less time involved scoring it.

Summary

Textbooks and semester courses have been dedicated to the science of psychometrics. The intent of this chapter has been to serve as a working outline for your reference, clarification, and repeated use to ensure that the scales you choose comprise the proper validity and reliability so you can confidently assess and report your patients' progress. We hope that these pages will become well-worn and dog-eared over time.

There is very little need for you to create your own measure when so many good, valid, easy-to-use, and free measures have already gone through the rigors of psychometric testing. As the field of MBC continues to grow, so will our psychological measurement vernacular. Speaking similar languages of psychiatric symptom scales keeps us on the same page, especially when collaborating with other professionals in the field, potential referrals, and our various stakeholders. Use what's out there; most of it is pretty good.

Chapter 06

Psychometric Test Access and User Qualifications

HAVING identified the measures you want to use in your measurement-based care (MBC) program, it is advisable to ensure that you can use those tools *without infringing on the copyrights of the test developer(s)*. Although many symptom rating scales and mental health measures are freely available, the onus for obtaining permission to use them (or for locating published statements that directly state unrestricted use is permitted) rests squarely on your shoulders.

Public Domain, Copyrighted, or Both?

Psychometric tests typically fall into two categories, those that are "free" and those that are not. The quotation marks around "free" is intentional because the line between freely available and copyrighted for some measures in the public domain can be a moving target. This is largely due to copyright laws and the natural evolution of the field. A measure that starts out as freely available in the public domain can later become a "commercial use only" tool (i.e., fee-based). The Mini-Mental State Examination (MMSE; Folstein et al. 1975) is a case in point (Fiore 2015). A preferred, brief cognitive screen used for decades by psychiatrists, psychologists, and neurologists alike, the MMSE's copyright was transferred to a commercial-use assessment company in 2001. Thus, its decades-long "free" use in both research and clinical realms came to a screeching halt.

The case of the MMSE is (we hope) an unusual, unique outcome, but it should give us pause and inspire reflection regarding what "copyright" means. Copyright laws are there to protect our rights as creators of sourced work, and these are automatically instated when a product is published. With respect to MBC, this means any symptom rating scale or quality-of-life measurement you choose for gauging therapeutic progress was copyrighted by its creator the moment it was published in the literature. These protections make sense because developing a test and validating it through scientific rigor is substantial dedicated work; test developers not only should be credited for their innovation but also deserve to have those products. Hays et al. (2018) elegantly stated that psychometrically sound tests are "the cornerstones of research and clinical assessment" (p. 6). The copyright means that the developer holds exclusive rights over the work and the power to permit others to use, distribute, or augment it, with or without payment.

In most academic circles, the spirit of sharing information and advancing the scientific and clinical field is a guiding force. Many test developers expect their work to be used freely for this purpose. But for an instrument to be used freely in the public domain, test developers must *actively notify users that they have waived the copyright protection for this purpose*. This is where the caution sign should grow larger. Even though the measure you choose is freely available in the public domain, this does not always mean that you can use it without obtaining permission. Part of the implementation process in your practice should include solidifying permission to use a particular measure. If you cannot identify a release statement in any of the publications, then simply emailing or contacting the lead author directly to obtain permission is a respectful, straightforward approach. In many instances, test developers appreciate the connection because they want to keep track of how their scales are being used and provide advice on proper administration (Hays et al. 2018).

Restricted Use

Most measures necessary to establish a clinically meaningful and psychometrically sound MBC program should be found and available in the public domain. Nevertheless, psychological tests that could be used for MBC also are available commercially and only through restricted access. These types of measures are restricted for very good reasons, many of which are attributed to the specialized advanced training within the domain of professional psychology. In Part I we said that MBC and psychological testing are not the same thing. The field of psychological assessment requires advanced training and expertise to provide comprehensive approaches for diagnosis, treatment recommendations, and deeper understanding of various mental health conditions. Measures designed to dig deeper, for instance, to rule out

TABLE 6–1.　Restricted use classifications for test user qualifications

Classification level	Qualifications of users
A	No special qualifications required for purchase, although range of availability is limited
B	Advance degree with knowledge of psychometrics and competencies in ethical use of tests required for purchase
C	Doctoral degree with demonstrated training in the administration and interpretation of psychological tests required for purchase

psychopathology, autism, or dementia, are those often exclusively available through restricted access. Further discussion here primarily provides clarity about how this is organized, thus saving you from barking up the wrong proverbial tree.

A fundamental principle guiding the restricted use of psychological tests is that only individuals with the appropriate training and expertise to administer, score, and interpret the tests may use them (American Educational Research Association et al. 2014). Restricting access ensures protection of the test, such as upholding its validity, protecting confidential scoring procedures, and reducing false diagnoses (Institute of Medicine 2015). In accordance with the American Psychological Association's *Guidelines for Test User Qualifications* (Turner et al. 2001), testing publishers such as Psychological Assessment Resources (www.parinc.com/Support/Qualification-Levels) and Pearson (www.pearsonassessments.com/professional-assessments/ordering/how-to-order/qualifications/qualifications-policy.html) typically use a three-pronged approach to classify the tests available for purchase based on the buyer's qualifications. Table 6–1 roughly summarizes these general classifications.

Summary

Albeit this is the shortest chapter in this book, it pulls its weight by expressing the formidable message that you must acquire the proper approvals for using the scales you have chosen. Additionally, it is crucial to ensure that any commercial online service you may hire has also garnered these necessary approvals, especially with respect to obtaining permission to transform valid measures into an electronic format. The little added effort to secure permission at the onset will not only save time in the long run but will also prevent any potential angst associated with copyright infringement.

Psychometrically Sound Scales

THIS chapter is assessment material heavy, presenting various resources for exploring, considering, and choosing measures that align with your practice mission, orientation, and business model. It is organized into three sections: "Open-Access Resources," "Commercial Packages," and "Psychiatric Symptom Scales." The presentation of these resources is extensive but not comprehensive. We do not represent ourselves as the sole authority for use of any of the measures nor for any of the available Web links from which to garner measurement-based care (MBC) measures. We encourage you to properly investigate each resource to ensure the test construction meets the standards of accepted validity and reliability and aligns with your own practice objectives.

Open-Access Resources

Several of the institutions listed in this chapter promote the implementation of MBC and thus have provided access to a compilation of measures from which clinicians may choose. These open-source resource websites are described, with their current Web addresses included.

American Psychiatric Association

DSM-5 Online Assessment Measures

www.psychiatry.org/psychiatrists/practice/dsm/ educational-resources/assessment-measures. To expand the traditional categorical practice of diagnosis, the DSM-5 Task Force introduced the use of dimensional assessments into the fifth edition of DSM (American Psychiatric Association 2013; Jones 2012). The conventional "Yes/No" categorical diagnostic process approached mental disorders as discrete phenomena, assuming pathology as homogeneous. Several researchers challenged the categorical approach to diagnosis as problematic because most patients present with wide-ranging comorbidities, thus recognizing the heterogeneous nature of mental health (Widiger and Coker 2003). Therefore, the implementation of dimensional—or cross-cutting—assessments into DSM-5 allowed diagnostic classification to exist along a continuum (Jones 2012; Widiger 2005). The categorical model is binary, whereas the dimensional model considers mental disorders to exist along a continuum of pathology. The tests selected by the DSM-5 Task Force, referred to as "emerging measures," account for the dimensional nature of mental conditions by having patients rate symptoms on scales signifying severity, intensity, frequency, and duration (Jones 2012), and most are compiled from the National Institutes of Health's Patient-Reported Outcomes Measurement Information System (PROMIS). The administration is a two-level approach. The first level requires patients to complete self-report measures, and if any domain is rated as clinically significant, the clinician then completes the level-two clinician-rated follow-up measures to provide more detailed assessment of the presenting condition. DSM-5 measures also should be administered to all patients at the initial evaluation to establish a baseline and subsequently throughout treatment to monitor patient progress, which is in line with MBC principles.

Mental Health Performance Measures

www.psychiatry.org/psychiatrists/practice/quality-improvement/ mental-health-performance-measures. This spreadsheet, compiled by American Psychiatric Association staff, is available on the psychiatry.org website to provide a comprehensive collection of mental health measures. The measures were compiled by accessing several measure databases, including the National Quality Measures Clearing House, the Center for Quality Assessment and Improvement in Mental Health, the National Quality Forum, and the Physicians Consortium for Performance Improvement. Each measure in the spreadsheet is categorized by diagnostic category and whether it is appropriate for use by care providers.

National Institutes of Health

Patient-Reported Outcomes Measurement Information System (PROMIS)

https://commonfund.nih.gov/promis. The National Institutes of Health's Roadmap for Medical Research initiative was launched in 2014 to support advances in medical science and translating research into practice (Kantor 2008). Part of this initiative was the development of PROMIS to develop valid self-report measures of health-related quality-of-life symptoms (Cella et al. 2010). PROMIS has since become a publicly available repository of valid and reliable measurement tools for providers' use to evaluate and monitor a wide age range of patients. The PROMIS repository offers a collection of medical, health, and mental health domains and related subdomains along with scoring manuals and related publications on validity. Some PROMIS tools can also be found in DSM's "emerging measures" repository.

RAND Corporation

Health Care Surveys

www.rand.org/health-care/surveys_tools.html. The RAND corporation (which is an acronym for Research and Development) offers a repository of freely available public domain measures on its website. Many of the scales can be used to measure treatment progress and outcomes and comprise categories such as general health and illness, mental health conditions, and quality of life. RAND researchers collaborated in the Medical Outcomes Study to develop cost effective ways to determine treatment effectiveness as it pertains to health-related quality of life (Tarlov et al. 1989). The construct of health-related quality of life is a recognized outcome across medical, epidemiological, and psychiatric care to gauge overall treatment effectiveness.

The Joint Commission

Chart Abstracted Measure Specifications Manuals

manual.jointcommission.org/bhcinstruments/webhome. As part of their effort to advance the Outcome Measures Standard CTS 03.01.09 to promote quality of mental health treatment through MBC, The Joint Commission created a resource page on their website listing standardized psychological instruments for accreditees to use to meet the new standard. Per their disclaimer, the provided list of psychological tests is neither endorsed nor promoted as an exclusive collection; consumers are encouraged to use their discretion when selecting from the repository.

MedWorks Media
Psychiatric Rating Scales

medworksmedia.com/product-category/rating-scales. MedWorks Media is a publisher of science education journals and special educational projects for psychiatrists, psychopharmacologists, and the larger medical community. Founded in 1994 by Dr. James La Rossa to promote the integration of clinical practice with psychiatric medicine, the website's resource link offers several validated psychiatric rating scales that are freely available for use in clinical practice. These include links to supporting validity studies in addition to manuals ranging from quality-of-life functioning to specific psychiatric symptom differentiation.

Psych Congress Network
Saundra's Corner

www.hmpgloballearningnetwork.com/site/pcn/ saundras-corner. Dr. Saundra Jain, motivated by the underuse of psychometric screeners as part of the therapeutic process, created a website toolbox of psychiatric rating scales to improve patient outcomes. As a proponent of MBC and successful outcomes, Dr. Jain provided a short list of accessible and well-known symptom scales that are freely available for download, including validity and reliability information as well as manuals for scoring.

Psychology Tools
Psychological Assessment Tools
for Mental Health

www.psychologytools.com/download-scales-and-measures. Founded by clinical psychologists in 2008, Psychology Tools is a resource library comprising evidenced-based scales and measures for mental health clinicians to use in conducting effective therapy. The compendium is organized intuitively for practitioners to navigate and find relevant measures for symptom assessment and practice outcomes. The website also serves as a resource for information on evidenced-based therapies and techniques, as well as summary articles written by their members.

Commercial Packages

Four commercial MBC assessment tools are listed. These assessment packages encompass the collective standard approach for measuring treatment progress as outlined in Part II. Brief descriptions for each of the four commercially available progress outcomes packages are also included to consider whether these systems best suit your needs rather than creating your own "do it yourself" method.

McLean Hospital

Behavior and Symptoms Identification System Scale (BASIS)

www.ebasis.org/basis24. Development of the BASIS began in the 1980s to create a brief yet comprehensive measurement tool to assess outcomes from substance abuse or mental health treatment programs (Jerrell 2005). The BASIS-24 and its predecessor, the BASIS-32, are self-report questionnaires that capture the severity and frequency of mental health and substance use symptoms in addition to symptom-related functional difficulties (Idiculla and Eisen 2012).

The BASIS-32 measures change in self-reported symptom and functional difficulty over the course of treatment and is purported to yield transdiagnostic indicators. It produces an overall score in addition to five subscales specific to domains of substance abuse and certain psychiatric symptoms: 1) Relation to Self and Others, 2) Depression and Anxiety, 3) Daily Living and Role Functioning, 4) Impulsive and Addictive Behavior, and 5) Psychosis.

The BASIS-24 was a revision to the BASIS-32 comprising a shorter version with improved reliability and validity in addition to expanding its validity for use in a greater diversity of patients (Eisen et al. 2004). Like its predecessor, the BASIS-24 assesses the degree of severity and frequency of mental health and substance use issues, yielding a revised set of six subscales: 1) Depression/Functioning, 2) Relationships, 3) Self-Harm, 4) Emotional Lability, 5) Psychosis, and 6) Substance Abuse. Reported psychometrics indicate excellent internal consistency (ranging from 0.75 to 0.91) and large Cronbach's α values in ethnic and gender subsamples (Idiculla and Eisen 2012).

BASIS scales are copyrighted and therefore require a site license obtained with an annual fee through McLean Hospital. The license offers several "levels" of use, ranging from independent and self-scoring use to membership in their Web-based community, called eBASIS, to receive aggregated reporting and Web-based services. You can integrate a paper-and-pencil version of the BASIS into your existing MBC infrastructure or access the BASIS entirely online.

Partners for Change Outcome Management System

Better Outcomes Now

www.betteroutcomesnow.com. Better Outcomes Now is the Web application of the Partners for Change Outcome Management System, created by Dr. Barry L. Duncan. Per their website, Better Outcomes Now combines science, technology, and clinical expertise to improve therapy outcomes by increasing information efficiency and supporting collaborative treatment decision-making. This approach uses its software, which includes the Session Rating Scale and Outcomes Rating Scale, to identify patients who are not responding well to therapy. It does so by addressing patients' lack of progress in a proactive way to keep them engaged while providers collaboratively seek new directions. Progress data are obtained for each clinical encounter that yield objective, quantifiable information on the therapeutic process.

Obtained with an annual subscription, Better Outcomes Now provides accurate, noninflated analysis of treatment effectiveness. It is designed with the nuances of the Partners for Change Outcome Management System clinical process in mind, as well the practicalities of both supervision and data analysis for quality improvement and reporting purposes.

Outcome Questionnaire Measures

Measure of Mental Health Vital Signs for Private Practices

www.oqmeasures.com. The Measure of Mental Health Vital Signs website is home to the Outcome Questionnaire (OQ) system. Unlike most psychological symptom measures, the OQ was developed primarily as a process and outcome measure to quantify and evaluate mental and behavioral health progress during therapy (Lambert et al. 1996). Most behavioral health questionnaires assess for specific symptoms, and most psychological assessments assign diagnoses, but the OQ measures are uniquely designed to track change over time during the course of psychotherapy. The OQ has been modified throughout the years, from the original OQ.45 to the newer OQ 45.2 version; subsequently, the program has broadened its scope to determine progress among severely mentally ill patients and track for psychological distress. It has also expanded to assess for therapeutic change in children and adolescents and for group psychotherapeutic progress.

The OQ-45.2 purports to measure therapeutic progress across three domains of subjective experience: 1) symptom distress, a subscale summarizing the degree of subjective discomfort; 2) interpersonal relations, a subscale regarding reported impairment in interpersonal functioning; and 3) social role, a subscale specific to assessing impairment in work and social functioning. Not only do OQ Measures track change during treatment, but the system also enlists a proprietary algorithm "alert" program to notify therapists about patient-specific rates of change. As described in Part II, these alerts are color-coded, ranging from white (patient is on track) to red (patient is worsening and at risk for dropout). The impetus behind OQ Measures is to detect negative outcomes prior to treatment failure in order to avoid that failure (Lambert 2010). One of Michael Lambert's major contributions was teaching us that providing feedback to therapists, especially when patients are not progressing therapeutically, reduces the likelihood of treatment failure. The OQ Measures program aims to maximize treatment effectiveness.

Outcome Referrals

The Treatment Outcome Package (TOP)

www.outcomereferrals.com/main/sub-page/category/ top-assessment. The TOP is a proprietary, multidimensional global assessment and treatment outcomes tool that measures the presence and severity of a wide range of behavioral health problems. Since its inception in the 1990s, it has undergone extensive psychometric rigor and analyses to establish its applicability for use in children, adolescents, and adults. For each age cohort assessment, it yields clinical and functional domains ranging from mood disorders and substance use to attention deficits and psychological strengths. Norms were established using both clinical and general populations, with strong test-retest reliability (0.76–0.94) and excellent discriminant, convergent, and predictive validity (Boswell et al. 2015; Kraus 2012).

The TOP is an MBC instrument intended for initial assessment followed by subsequent administrations. It can be completed using paper-and-pencil methods or online. As a fee-for-service product, one of its offerings includes patented technology to produce customized reminder links for patients to complete the TOP within the prescribed time intervals (thereby saving precious therapy time by having them complete the assessment at home). Another service benefit is the multipage feedback report the system provides after each administration to demonstrate patient progress; included in this output are designated "alerts" when patients are not on track, along with accompanied tailored resource suggestions to support treatment success (Kraus et al. 2006).

The TOP assessment is one of the services offered through the Outcomes Referrals group. As the company grows, so does its advancements in offering innovative solutions for behavioral health management, such as the use of artificial intelligence to predict behavioral health risk indicators in patients and to successfully match therapist to patient through its algorithms.

Psychiatric Symptom Scales

Table 7–1 lists an ample compendium of public-domain, free-access measures. The measures are listed in alphabetical order by psychiatric diagnosis and include the test's parent article citation to promote further examination of its appropriateness for your use. Some sections are further organized by age cohort.

Most of these scales are found in the public domain and free to use. As outlined in Part III, it is your responsibility to obtain the required permission to use any measure that does not clearly denote copyright waiver. Not all reference articles display conspicuous statements releasing copyright. Therefore, proceed with caution, obtain permission when necessary, and print out release statements (whether from the measurement website or an email from the developer); keep these printed notices in the same folder that holds your compilation of journal articles justifying the use of your chosen measure.

TABLE 7–1. Psychiatric symptom scales alphabetized by disorder

Scales	Citation	Acronym	Items, N
Anxiety (adult)			
Clinically Useful Anxiety Outcome Scale	Zimmerman M, Chelminski I, Young D, et al: A clinically useful anxiety outcome scale. J Clin Psychiatry 71(5):534–542, 2010	CUXOS	20
Fear Questionnaire	Van Zuuren FJ: The Fear Questionnaire: some data on validity, reliability and layout. Br J Psychiatry 153:659–662, 1988	FQ	24
Generalized Anxiety Disorder Screener	Spitzer RL, Kroenke K, Williams JB, et al: A brief measure for assessing generalized anxiety disorder: the GAD-7. Arch Intern Med 166(10):1092–1097, 2006	GAD-7	7
Hamilton Rating Scale for Anxiety	Hamilton M: The assessment of anxiety states by rating. Br J Med Psychol 32(1):50–55, 1959	HAM-A	15
Liebowitz Social Anxiety Scale	Liebowitz MR: Social phobia. Mod Probl Pharmacopsychiatry 22:141–173, 1987	LSAS-SR	24
Panic Disorder Severity Scale	Shear MK, Brown TA, Barlow DH, et al: Multicenter collaborative panic disorder severity scale. Am J Psychiatry 154(11):1571–1575, 1997	PDSS-SR	7
Penn State Worry Questionnaire	Meyer TJ, Miller ML, Metzger RL, et al: Development and validation of the Penn State Worry Questionnaire. Behav Res Ther 28(6):487–495, 1990	PSWQ	16
Social Phobia Inventory	Connor KM, Davidson JR, Churchill LE, et al: Psychometric properties of the Social Phobia Inventory (SPIN): new self-rating scale. Br J Psychiatry 176:379–386, 2000	SPIN	17

TABLE 7–1. Psychiatric symptom scales alphabetized by disorder (*continued*)

Scales	Citation	Acronym	Items, N
Anxiety (youth)			
Penn State Worry Questionnaire for Children	Chorpita BF, Tracey SA, Brown TA, et al: Assessment of worry in children and adolescents: an adaptation of the Penn State Worry Questionnaire. Behav Res Ther 35(6):569–581, 1997	PSWQ-C	14
Revised Children's Anxiety and Depression Scale Youth	Chorpita BF, Yim LM, Moffitt CE, et al: Assessment of symptoms of DSM-IV anxiety and depression in children: a revised child anxiety and depression scale. Behav Res Ther 38(8):835–855, 2000	RCADS	47
Screen for Child Anxiety Related Emotion Disorders	Birmaher B, Brent DA, Chiappetta L, et al: Psychometric properties of the Screen for Child Anxiety Related Emotional Disorders (SCARED): a replication study. J Am Acad Child Adolesc Psychiatry 38(10):1230–1236, 1999	SCARED	41
Spence Children's Anxiety Scale	Spence SH: A measure of anxiety symptoms among children. Behav Res Ther 36(5):545–566, 1998	SCAS	44
Attention-deficit/hyperactivity disorder (ADHD)			
Strengths and Weaknesses of Attention-Deficit/Hyperactivity Symptoms and Normal Behaviors	Young DA, Levy F, Martin NC, et al: Attention-deficit hyperactivity disorder: a Rasch analysis of the SWAN Rating Scale. Child Psychiatry Hum Dev 40(4):543–559, 2009	SWAN	18
Swanson Nolan and Pelham questionnaire	Hall CL, Guo B, Valentine AZ, et al: The validity of the SNAP-IV in children displaying ADHD symptoms. Assessment 27(6):1258–1271, 2020	SNAP-IV	26

TABLE 7-1. Psychiatric symptom scales alphabetized by disorder (*continued*)

Scales	Citation	Acronym	Items, *N*
ADHD (*continued*)			
Vanderbilt ADHD Rating Scale	Wolraich M, Lambert MJ, Doffing M, et al: Psychometric properties of the Vanderbilt ADHD Diagnostic Parent Rating Scale in a referred population. J Pediatr Psychol 28(8):559–568, 2003	VADRS	26
Autism			
Autism-Spectrum Quotient Test	Baron-Cohen S, Wheelwright S, Skinner R, et al: The Autism-spectrum Quotient (AQ): evidence from Asperger syndrome/high-functioning autism, males and females, scientists and mathematicians. J Autism Dev Disord 31(1):5–17, 2001	AQ	50
Empathy Quotient	Baron-Cohen S, Wheelwright S: The Empathy Quotient: an investigation of adults with Asperger syndrome or high functioning autism, and normal sex differences. J Autism Dev Disord 34(2):163–175, 2004	EQ	60
Modified Checklist for Autism in Toddlers	Robins DL, Fein D, Barton ML, et al: The Modified Checklist for Autism in Toddlers: an initial study investigating the early detection of autism and pervasive developmental disorders. J Autism Dev Disord 31(2):131–144, 2001	M-CHAT	23
Behavioral problems (youth)			
Disruptive Behavior Child and Adolescent Inventory–Parent and Teacher	Cianchetti C, Pittau A, Carta V, et al: Child and Adolescent Behavior Inventory (CABI): a new instrument for epidemiological studies and pre-clinical evaluation. Clin Pract Epidemiol Ment Health 9:51–61, 2013	CABI	25

TABLE 7–1.   Psychiatric symptom scales alphabetized by disorder (continued)

Scales	Citation	Acronym	Items, N
Behavioral problems (youth) *(continued)*			
Disruptive Behavior Disorders Rating Scale	Silva RR, Alpert M, Pouget E, et al: A rating scale for disruptive behavior disorders, based on the DSM-IV item pool. Psychiatr Q 76(4):327–339, 2005	DBDRS	45
Strengths and Difficulties Questionnaire	Richter J: The Strengths and Difficulties Questionnaire (SDQ). Eur Child Adolesc Psychiatry 12:1–8, 2003	SDQ	25
Youth Top Problems	Weisz JR, Chorpita BF, Frye A, et al: Youth Top Problems: using idiographic, consumer-guided assessment to identify treatment needs and to track change during psychotherapy. J Consult Clin Psychol 79(3):369–380, 2011	TP	11
Bipolar/Mania (adult)			
Altman Self-Rating Mania Scale	Hedeker D: The Altman Self-Rating Mania Scale. Biol Psychiatry 42:948–955, 1997	ASRAM	5
Bech–Rafaelsen Mania Scale	Bech P, Bolwig TG, Kramp P, et al: The Bech–Rafaelsen Mania Scale and the Hamilton Depression Scale. Acta Psychiatr Scand 59(4):420–430, 1979	MAS	11
Mood Disorder Questionnaire	Hirschfeld R, Williams J, Spitzer RL, et al: Development and validation of a screening instrument for bipolar spectrum disorder: the Mood Disorder Questionnaire. Am J Psychiatry 157(11):1873–1875, 2000	MDQ	17
Young Mania Rating Scale	Young RC, Biggs JT, Ziegler VE, et al: A rating scale for mania: reliability, validity and sensitivity. Br J Psychiatry 133:429–435, 1978	YMRS	11

TABLE 7–1. Psychiatric symptom scales alphabetized by disorder *(continued)*

Scales	Citation	Acronym	Items, N
Bipolar/Mania (youth)			
Child Mania Rating Scale–Parent	Pavuluri MN, Henry DB, Devineni B, et al: Child Mania Rating Scale: development, reliability, and validity. J Am Acad Child Adolesc Psychiatry 45(5):550–560, 2006	CMRS-P	21
Parent Version of the Young Mania Rating Scale	Marchand WR, Clark SC, Wirth L, et al: Validity of the parent Young Mania Rating Scale in a community mental health setting. Psychiatry (Edgmont) 2(3):31–35, 2005	P-YMRS	11
Depression (adult)			
Center for Epidemiologic Studies Depression Scale	Radloff LS: The CES-D scale: a self-report depression scale for research in the general population. Appl Psychol Meas 1(3):385–401, 1977	CES-D	20
Clinically Useful Depression Outcome Scale	Zimmerman M, Chelminski I, McGlinchey JB, et al: A clinically useful depression outcome scale. Compr Psychiatry 49(2):131–140, 2007	CUDOS	18
Hamilton Rating Scale for Depression	Hamilton MA: A rating scale for depression. J Neurol Neurosurg Psychiatry 23(1):56–62, 1960	HAM-D	17
The Inventory of Depressive Symptoms	Rush AJ, Giles DE, Schlesser MA, et al: The Inventory for Depressive Symptomatology (IDS): preliminary findings. Psychiatry Res 18(1):65–87, 1986	IDS	30
Kessler Psychiatric Distress Scale	Kessler RC, Andrews G, Colpe LJ, et al: Short screening scales to monitor population prevalences and trends in non-specific psychological distress. Psychol Med 32(6):959–976, 2002	K-10	10

TABLE 7–1.   Psychiatric symptom scales alphabetized by disorder (continued)

Scales	Citation	Acronym	Items, N
Depression (adult) (continued)			
Major Depression Inventory	Olsen LR, Jensen DV, Noerholm V, et al: The internal and external validity of the Major Depression Inventory in measuring severity of depressive states. Psychol Med 33:351–356, 2003	MDI	10
Patient Health Questionnaire–9	Kroenke K, Spitzer RL, Williams JBW: The PHQ-9: validity of a brief depression severity measure. J Gen Intern Med 16(9):606–613, 2001	PHQ-9	9
Quick Inventory of Depressive Symptomatology	Rush AJ, Trivedi MH, Ibrahim HM, et al: The 16-item Quick Inventory of Depressive Symptomatology (QIDS), Clinician Rating (QIDS-C), and Self-Report (QIDS-SR): a psychometric evaluation in patients with chronic major depression. Biol Psychiatry 54(5):573–583, 2003	QIDS-SR	16
Depression (youth)			
Center for Epidemiologic Studies Depression Scale for Children	Radloff LS: The use of the Center for Epidemiologic Studies Depression Scale in adolescents and young adults. J Youth Adolesc 20(2):149–166, 1991	CES-DC	20
Children's Revised Impact of Event Scale	Perrin S, Meiser-Stedman R, Smith P: The Children's Revised Impact of Event Scale (CRIES): validity as a screening instrument for PTSD. Behav Cogn Psychother 33(4):487–498, 2005	CRIES	13
Depression Self Rating Scale for Children	Birelson P: The validity of depressive disorder in childhood and the development of a self-rating scale: a research report. J Psychol Psychiatry 22(1):73–88, 1981	DSRSC	18

TABLE 7–1. Psychiatric symptom scales alphabetized by disorder *(continued)*

Scales	Citation	Acronym	Items, N
Depression (youth) *(continued)*			
Kutcher Adolescent Depression Scale	Brooks SJ, Krulewicz SP, Kutcher S: The Kutcher Adolescent Depression Scale: assessment of its evaluative properties over the course of an 8-week pediatric pharmacotherapy trial. J Child Adolesc Psychopharmacol 13(3):337–349, 2003	KADS	11
Mood and Feelings Questionnaire	Costello EJ, Angold A: Scales to assess child and adolescent depression: checklists, screens, and nets. J Am Acad Child Adolesc Psychiatry 27(6):726–737, 1988	MFQ	33
Patient Health Questionnaire–Adolescent	Johnson JG, Harris ES, Spitzer RL, et al: The Patient Health Questionnaire for Adolescents: validation of an instrument for the assessment of mental disorders among adolescent primary care patients. J Adolesc Health 30(3):196–204, 2002	PHQ-A	9
Short Mood and Feelings Questionnaire	Thapar A, McGuffin P: Validity of the shortened Mood and Feelings Questionnaire in a community sample of children and adolescents: a preliminary research note. Psychiatry Res 81(2):259–268, 1998	SMFQ	13
Eating disorders			
Child Eating Attitudes Test	Smolak L, Levine MP: Psychometric properties of the Children's Eating Attitudes Test. Int J Eat Disord 16(3):275–282, 1994	ChEAT	26
Eating Attitudes Test-26	Garner DM, Olmsted MP, Bohr Y, et al: The Eating Attitudes Test: psychometric features and clinical correlates. Psychol Med 12(4):871–878, 1982	EAT-26	26

TABLE 7–1. Psychiatric symptom scales alphabetized by disorder *(continued)*

Scales	Citation	Acronym	Items, N
Medication side effects and adherence			
Frequency, Intensity, Burden of Side Effects Rating Scale	Wisniewski SR, Rush AJ, Balasubramani GK, et al: Self-rated global measure of the frequency, intensity and burden of side effects. J Psychiatr Practice 12(2):71–79, 2006	FIBSER	3
Glasgow Antipsychotics Side Effect Scale	Waddell L, Taylor M: A new self-rating scale for detecting atypical or second-generation antipsychotic side effects. J Psychopharmacol 22(3):238–243, 2008	GASS	22
Liverpool University Neuroleptic Side-Effect Rating Scale	Day JC, Wood G, Dewey M, et al: A self-rating scale for measuring neuroleptic side-effects: validation in a group of schizophrenic patients. Br J Psychiatry 166(5):650–653, 1995	LUNSERS	41
Systematic Monitoring of Adverse events Related to TreatmentS	Haddad PM, Fleischhacker WW, Peuskens J, et al: SMARTS (Systematic Monitoring of Adverse events Related to TreatmentS): the development of a pragmatic patient-completed checklist to assess antipsychotic drug side effects. Ther Adv Psychopharmacol 4(1):15–21, 2014	SMARTS	11
Obsessive-compulsive disorder			
Children's Yale-Brown Obsessive Compulsive Scale	Scahill L, Riddle MA, McSwiggin-Hardin M, et al: Children's Yale-Brown Obsessive Compulsive Scale: reliability and validity. J Am Acad Child Adolesc Psychiatry 36(6):844–852, 1997	CY-BOCS	19
Yale-Brown Obsessive Compulsive Scale	Goodman WK, Price LH, Rasmussen SA, et al: The Yale-Brown Obsessive Compulsive Scale, I: development, use, and reliability. Arch Gen Psychiatry 46(11):1006–1011, 1989	Y-BOCS	10+

TABLE 7–1. Psychiatric symptom scales alphabetized by disorder *(continued)*

Scales	Citation	Acronym	Items, N
PTSD (adult)			
Impact of Event Scale–Revised	Weiss DS: The Impact of Event Scale–Revised, in Cross-Cultural Assessment of Psychological Trauma and PTSD (International and Cultural Psychology Series). Edited by Wilson JP, Tang CS. Boston, MA, Springer, 2007, pp 219–238	IES-R	22
Los Angeles Symptom Checklist	King LA, King DW, Leskin G, et al: The Los Angeles Symptom Checklist: a self report measure of post-traumatic stress disorder. Assessment 2(1):1–17, 1995	LASC	43
Post-Traumatic Stress Disorder Checklist–Civilian Version	Weathers FW, Litz BT, Keane TM, et al: The PTSD Checklist for DSM-5 (PCL-5). 2013. Available at: www.ptsd.va.gov/professional/assessment/adult-sr/ptsd-checklis-.asp#obtain. Accessed January 6, 2022.	PCL-C	17
Trauma History Questionnaire	Hooper L, Stockton P, Krupnick J, et al: Development, use, and psychometric properties of the Trauma History Questionnaire. J Loss Trauma 16(3):258–283, 2011	THQ	24
Trauma History Screen	Carlson EB, Smith SR, Palmieri PA, et al: Development and validation of a brief self-report measure of trauma exposure: the Trauma History Screen. Psychol Assess 23(2):463–477, 2011	THS	14
PTSD (youth)			
Child PTSD Symptom Scale	Foa EB, Johnson KM, Feeny NC, et al: The Child PTSD Symptom Scale: a preliminary examination of its psychometric properties. J Clin Child Psychol 30(3):376–384, 2001	CPSS	17

TABLE 7–1.　Psychiatric symptom scales alphabetized by disorder *(continued)*

Scales	Citation	Acronym	Items, *N*
PTSD (youth) *(continued)*			
Pediatric Emotional Distress Scale	Saylor CF, Swenson CC, Reynolds SS, et al: The Pediatric Emotional Distress Scale: a brief screening measure for young children exposed to traumatic events. J Clin Child Psychol 28(1):70–81, 1999	PEDS	21
Quality of life (adult)			
Daily Living Activities Scale	Roger S, Presmanes W: Reliability and validity of the Daily Living Activities Scale: a functional assessment measure for severe mental disorders. Res Soc Work Pract 11(3):373–389, 2001	DLA-20	20
Functional Outcomes Survey–20	Stewart A, Hays R, Ware J: The MOS short-form general health survey: reliability and validity in a patient population. Med Care 26(7):724–735, 1988	SF-20	20
World Health Organization Disability Assessment Schedule 2.0	Üstün TB, Chatterji S, Kostanjsek N, et al: Developing the World Health Organization Disability Assessment Schedule 2.0. Bull World Health Organ 88(11):815–823, 2010	WHODAS 2.0	36
World Health Organization Quality of Life	Skevington SM, Lotfy M, O'Connell KA: The World Health Organization's WHOQOL-BREF quality of life assessment: psychometric properties and results of the international field trial: a report from the WHOQOL group. Quality of Life Research 13(2):299–310, 2004	WHOQOL	26

TABLE 7–1. Psychiatric symptom scales alphabetized by disorder *(continued)*

Scales	Citation	Acronym	Items, N
Quality of life (youth)			
Brief Impairment Scale	Bird HR, Canino GJ, Davies M, et al: The Brief Impairment Scale (BIS): a multidimensional scale of functional impairment for children and adolescents. J Am Acad Child Adolesc Psychiatry 44(7):699–707, 2005	BIS	24
Brief Problem Checklist	Chorpita BF, Reise S, Weisz JR, et al: Evaluation of the Brief Problem Checklist: child and caregiver interviews to measure clinical progress. J Consult Clin Psychol 78(4):526–536, 2010	BPC	12
Columbia Impairment Scale	Attell BK, Cappelli C, Manteuffel B, et al: Measuring functional impairment in children and adolescents: psychometric properties of the Columbia impairment Scale (CIS). Evaluation and the Health Professions 43(1):3–15, 2020	CIS	20
Ohio Scale for Youth	Ogles BM, Dowell K, Hatfield D, et al: The Ohio Scales, in The Use of Psychological Testing for Treatment Planning and Outcomes Assessment: Instruments for Children and Adolescents, Vol 2, 3rd Edition. Edited by Maruish ME. Hillsdale, NJ, Lawrence Erlbaum, 2004, pp 275–304	OSY	20
Peabody Treatment Progress Battery	Riemer M, Athay MM, Bickman L, et al. The Peabody Treatment Progress Battery: history and methods for developing a comprehensive measurement battery for youth mental health. Adm Policy Ment Health 39(1–2):3–12, 2012	PTPB	N/A
Pediatric Symptom Checklist–Youth	Blucker RT, Jackson D, Gillaspy JA, et al: Pediatric behavioral health screening in primary care: a preliminary analysis of the Pediatric Symptom Checklist-17 with functional impairment items. Clin Pediatr 53(5):449–455, 2014	Y-PSC	17

TABLE 7–1.   Psychiatric symptom scales alphabetized by disorder (*continued*)

Scales	Citation	Acronym	Items, N
Substance use			
Alcohol, Smoking and Substance Involvement Screening Test	WHO ASSIST Working Group: The Alcohol, Smoking and Substance Involvement Screening Test (ASSIST): development, reliability and feasibility. Addiction 97(9): 1183–1194, 2002	ASSIST	9
Alcohol Use Disorders Identification Test	Bohn MJ, Babor TF, Kranzler HR: The Alcohol Use Disorders Identification Test (AUDIT): validation of a screening instrument for use in medical settings. J Stud Alcohol 56(4):423–432, 1995	AUDIT-C	10
Brief Addiction Monitor	Cacciola JS, Alterman AI, DePhilippis D, et al: Development and initial evaluation of the Brief Addiction Monitor (BAM). J Subst Abuse Treat 44(3):256–263, 2013	BAM	17
Drug Abuse Screening Test	Skinner HA: The Drug Abuse Screening Test. Addict Behav 7(4):363–371, 1982	DAST-10	10
Suicidality			
Columbia Suicide Severity Rating Scale	Posner K, Brown GK, Stanley B, et al: The Columbia Suicide Severity Rating Scale: initial validity and internal consistency findings from three multisite studies with adolescents and adults. Am J Psychiatry 168:1266–1277, 2011	C-SSRS	20
Suicide Behaviors Questionnaire–Revised	Rueda-Jaimes GE, Castro-Rueda VA, Rangel-Martínez-Villalba AM, et al: Validity of the Suicide Behaviors Questionnaire–Revised in patients with short-term suicide risk. Eur J Psychiatry 31(4):145–150, 2017	SBQ-R	4

TABLE 7–1. Psychiatric symptom scales alphabetized by disorder *(continued)*

Scales	Citation	Acronym	Items, *N*
Treatment alliance			
California Psychotherapy Alliance Scales	Delsignore A, Rufer M, Moergeli H, et al: California Psychotherapy Alliance Scale (CALPAS): psychometric properties of the German version for group and individual therapy patients. Compr Psychiatry 55(3):736–742, 2015	CALPAS	
Multidimensional Scale of Perceived Social Support	Dahlem NW, Zimet GD, Walker RR: The Multidimensional Scale of Perceived Social Support: a confirmation study. J Clin Psychol 47(6):756–761, 1991	MSPSS	32
Revised Helping Alliance Questionnaire	Luborsky L, Barber JP, Siqueland L, et al: The Revised Helping Alliance Questionnaire (HAq-II): psychometric properties. J Psychother Pract Res 5(3):260–271, 1996	HAq-II	19
Treatment progress and satisfaction			
Client Satisfaction Questionnaire	Attkisson CC, Zwick R: The Client Satisfaction Questionnaire: psychometric properties and correlations with service utilization and psychotherapy outcome. Eval Program Plann 5(3):233–237, 1982	CSQ-18	18
Stages of Change Scale	Gonzalez-Ramirez LP, De la Roca-Chiapas JM, Colunga-Rodriguez C, et al: Validation of Health Behavior and Stages of Change Questionnaire. Breast Cancer (Dove Med Press) 9:199–205, 2017	SCS	12
University of Rhode Island Change Assessment	Field CA, Adinoff B, Harris TR, et al: Construct, concurrent and predictive validity of the URICA: data from two multi-site clinical trials. Drug Alcohol Depend 101(1–2):115–123, 2009	URICA	24

PART IV

Aggregating Measurement-Based Care for Program Fidelity

Chapter 08

Aggregating Patient Data for Program Fidelity

THE primary objective of this book has been to serve the clinician, irrespective of professional acumen, to confidently implement and use measurement-based care (MBC) as part of the psychotherapeutic process. In many settings, especially community-based or large mental health facilities, aggregating patient MBC data provides opportunities to support quality assurance (QA) initiatives, substantiate treatment program fidelity, and establish a platform from which to report program effectiveness for various stakeholders. In this chapter, we provide a basic overview of the methods and applications of combining patient MBC data for these purposes.

Quality Assurance

The practice of assuring quality of care has been an enduring standard for medical services delivery and, more recently, mental health services delivery. The primary function of QA is to monitor the effectiveness of mental health services through an established program of oversight and audit, improving when needed and ensuring access to and receipt of quality care. The Institute of Medicine (2006) stipulated that implementing a QA (and quality improvement) practice was one of the most promising means to improved care. Furthermore, accrediting agencies require behavioral health programs to show that they use QA procedures.

Effective QA practices can verify program fidelity, identify gaps in programming, and determine patient satisfaction with services as well as substantiate the extent and benchmarks of clinical programming effectiveness. It is also useful for identifying unmet patient needs and ascertaining clinicians' areas of strength or weakness. QA factors are typically determined using the Donabedian classification system, which underpins the measurement system for quality improvement. These three component measures are structure, process, and outcome measures (Donabedian 1966).

MBC factors into QA and quality improvement methods by integrating patient progress data into the outcome measures component of the Donabedian system. The structure-measures component entails the physical and organizational components of service delivery, such as staff-to-patient ratio or clinical credentialing. The process-measures component includes issues such as treatment fidelity (i.e., whether overall care was delivered properly) and more detailed issues such as patient wait times. The outcome-measures component reflects the end result of treatment, such as the length of stay and the extent to which symptoms were reduced or treatment goals were met. The latter can be achieved through the aggregation and analysis of MBC data. According to Donabedian, outcome measures are the "ultimate validators" of treatment effectiveness and quality care, although all three components play necessary roles critical for comprehensive QA. Implementing MBC not only improves patients' therapeutic outcomes or the therapeutic alliance but also can easily extend to serve program fidelity management.

Building each patient's MBC data into an aggregated data bank will provide the foundation from which your MBC program's outcomes will tell the story of its overall effectiveness and support your QA mission.

Data Management Guidelines

Adhering to established guidelines is imperative for properly managing data in order to maintain its integrity and neutrality. Mental health data collected through MBC are not excluded from such standards. Reporting MBC outcomes for QA and site-specific dissemination may not require the same data management rigor as national grant-funded research, yet aggregating MBC data should still follow established guidelines from which to ensure best practices. Before implementing your MBC program, check with your institution's policy on psychological or clinical data management. If no guidelines have been established, consider consulting with an affiliated university for guidance in setting up such a data management system. Some universities, such as Columbia University, provide data management and analysis collaboration with affiliated mental health treatment centers.

Following established guidelines is an ounce of prevention. Thoroughly identifying the steps to aggregate MBC data tempers one's enthusiasm to dump everything into a data bank without much forethought. Depending on the clinic(s), aggregation of data must consider demographics, patients' presenting conditions and comorbidities, and treating clinicians' varying treatment plans and orientations. Without a plan to account for these variables, the resulting data analyses could produce incorrect and potentially harmful conclusions (Shamoo and Resnick 2009). Expect to have the data scrutinized, as they should be. As the field of MBC grows, so will "reported outcomes" publications. As members of the behavioral health industry, we should approach the methods and analyses of MBC with the same best-practices rigor and ethics as we do our clinical work. This will protect MBC as a burgeoning field and help it gain traction as a legitimate method of practice-based evidence. This chapter merely introduces considerations for ethical data management guidelines and the steps needed for practitioners to build their own programs to manage, clean, and report aggregated MBC data.

Building MBC Data

Part II outlined the basic steps for collecting MBC data specific to each patient. Simple stuff, in terms of data processing: patient completes a symptom scale, you score it, plot the summated score, and save the paper survey and data graphs in the patient's file. However, if one of your practice objectives is to report on overall program effectiveness, then building the data collection program at the onset of MBC implementation is proactive and can be accomplished with just a few extra steps. Hiring a commercial data analytics firm is a simple solution to building a data bank, but not all psychotherapeutic practices can afford such amenities. Nevertheless, a do-it-yourself approach to building your a data bank using a commercial or open-source spreadsheet program such as Microsoft Excel (www.microsoft.com) or LibreOffice Calc (www.libreoffice.org) is not only feasible and cost-effective but also manageable. Using a spreadsheet program serves many time-saving functions for data storage, data management, and basic calculations, not to mention reducing human calculation errors. Mastering basic strategies in an open-source spreadsheet program is nothing short of magical and will save immeasurable time in collecting, coding, and preparing data. Furthermore, data organized via spreadsheet programs will easily transfer into statistical software packages for more advanced analyses. The discussions that follow describe the management of MBC data using Microsoft Excel.

Organizing Data

We build our MBC data banks one patient at a time. Before the first patient's data are entered, however, we must establish the architecture of data organization. Like any spreadsheet, Excel and LibreOffice Calc are configured in columns and rows. At the top of each column a header can be assigned a variable (e.g., "name," "age," or "diagnosis") and each row assigned a patient. Organizing data in this linear fashion (in rows) allows the data bank fields to grow over time as more patients are entered. When the data are set up with one row per person (or "wide format"), the individual patient is the focus of the unit of analysis. For MBC, the first few column header titles should be for demographic information, such as the patient's name, date of birth, medical record number, and date of beginning therapy. Subsequent columns should be for each item from the symptom scales chosen for MBC. Figure 8–1 illustrates how a Microsoft Excel program could be formatted using Patient Health Questionnaire–9 (PHQ-9) data for this example.

In Figure 8–1, there are fields to capture the exact date on which the survey was completed. The temporal nature of MBC, and thus repeated administrations, necessitates logging the dates of testing administration. Furthermore, to organize this information cleanly, the date and all the data collected at that time should be denoted using the same prefix identifier. In the figure, the column labels denote a prefix identifier such as "Pre." and "Wk2." to indicate date and PHQ-9 scores taken at intake and at Week 2, respectively. Lastly, it is judicious practice to enter each item response in addition to the summated score; although subsequent aggregate analyses will rely primarily on summed scores, obtaining and saving original raw individual scores provides a framework for checks and double-checks. This includes correcting for missing data, double-checking score calculations, and allowing for item analysis should it be later warranted.

At this initial level of data capture, organizing data by actual patient name is essential to ensure that the right data are assigned to the right patient. After treatment termination, however, data should be moved into a treatment-complete data bank, and any identifying information, such as names, should be deidentified using numerical assignment to ensure privacy protection.

Coding Data

Each item response or answer option in the symptom scales used for MBC will almost always be assigned some type of numerical indicator, usually an assigned number based on test design. Answer options are best understood to comprise scales of measurement, falling under the N-O-I-R categories, representing nominal, ordinal, interval, and ratio scales (Stevens 1946). Nominal scale answer options do not have any intrinsic ordering to them and are best understood as labels, such as yes or no, gender identities, or levels of education. Ordinal scale answer choices represent meaningful ranking among the answer options and are often those used in public-domain symptom scales.

	A	B	C	D	E	F	G	H	I	J	K	L	M	N	O	P	Q	R
1	First name	Last name	Med rec#	Pre. date	Pre. PHQ1	Pre. PHQ2	Pre. PHQ3	Pre. PHQ4	Pre. PHQ5	Pre. PHQ6	Pre. PHQ7	Pre. PHQ8	Pre. PHQ9	Pre. PHQ.sum	Wk.2. date	Wk.2. PHQ1	Wk.2. PHQ2	Wk.2. PHQ3
2	John	Smith	1234	15-Jan	3	3	2	2	1	3	3	1	3	21	29-Jan	3	3	2
3	Jane	Doe	2345	19-Jan	2	2	3	3	3	3	2	2	3	23	2-Feb	2	2	2
4	David	Johnes	3456	20-Jan	3	2	3	3	2	1	1	3	2	20	3-Feb	3	2	3

FIGURE 8–1. Basic spreadsheet data bank formatting to capture measurement-based care, by patient, over time.

PHQ=Patient Health Questionnaire; Pre.=pre-treatment (intake); rec=record; Wk=week.

These represent the ubiquitous "on a scale from 1 to 10, where 10 is the best..." or the ever-popular Likert-type scale, which traditionally uses a five- to seven-item response scheme based on the assumption that the degree of responses is linear (Carifio and Perla 2007). These include capturing the intensity of an attitude, degree of agreement or satisfaction, or frequency of behavior, to name a few. Interval and ratio scales are very similar in construction; the distance between each answer option has meaning, for example, temperature and weight, respectively. The difference, however, is with respect to true zero. Temperature scales are interval because using 0° to describe how cold it is does not make much logical sense. "Zero" means the absence of something; therefore, there is no real 0° in weather. In weight, however, there is a true zero; something can realistically have absolutely no weight whatsoever. Therefore, weight scales are ratio, and temperature scales are interval.

In most instances, the scales you choose will already have coded responses assigned. Your job is to simply enter these data into your data base. Additional coding may come into play should you wish to add demographic and medical record health information, such as age, gender, education, or primary diagnosis. Many of these variables are categorical and will need to be assigned a nominal number code for each sub-designation within each category. To keep all the assigned coding designations organized, it is important to create a data dictionary, as denoted in Table 8–1. The data dictionary is a living document that captures all the measures used in MBC, along with a detailed outline of what each of the assigned answer options represents qualitatively. These come in handy when one needs to remember that a "5" on one scale does not necessarily correspond to a "5" on another.

Calculating Data

Before we can interpret the meaning of a psychological scale, we must first calculate each item score in some fashion based on scoring rules found in each test's manual. Many public-domain symptom scales are simply calculated by summing all the items into a "summary" score that can be done with a calculator or programmed to add the items using a calculation formula in an Excel spreadsheet. Returning to Figure 8–1, for example, we can simply add the nine items of the PHQ-9 to yield its summed score or code a formula in Excel to do the calculation for us. John Smith's intake summed PHQ-9 (see cell N2) can be a coded formula of "=SUM(E2:M2)" to yield his summated score of 21. Once this formula is copied into subsequent cells in that column (adjusting to account for the row designation), the added burden of having to sum every PHQ-9 has been removed. Beyond the summated calculations are other coding schemes, such as calculating subscales (e.g., the PTSD Checklist for DSM-5 illustrated in Chapter 3), identifying reverse-

TABLE 8–1. Sample data dictionary to illustrate assigned code per qualifier

Data dictionary		
Scale	**Code**	**Qualifier**
Education	1	Up through high school
	2	Up through undergraduate
	3	Postgraduate education
Presenting problem	1	Mood disorders
	2	Anxiety disorders
	3	Comorbid anxiety and mood
	4	Trauma and stress disorders
	5	Psychotic disorders
Patient Health Questionnaire–9	0	Not at all
	1	Several days
	2	More than half the days
	3	Nearly every day

code items and then calculating those scores based on the test's scoring manual, or transforming raw scores into *t*-scores. In each instance, it is necessary to read the symptom scale's test manual on scoring procedures in order to create a scoring cheat sheet for those requiring special coding (or program the Excel data bank to compute it for you).

Most of the scales that provide guidelines for transforming raw scores into *t*-scores include the *t*-score table in their scoring instructions. The *t*-score in psychological testing is a method to describe how a person compares with others on a normal distribution. The "mean" *t*-score is always 50, with a standard deviation of 10. In most psychological tests, a *t*-score ≥65 reflects modest difficulties, and ≥70 is considered problematic. Patient-Reported Outcomes Measurement Information System (PROMIS) scales almost always include the *t*-tables to aid in transforming the raw score to a *t*-score. Figure 8–2 illustrates the raw data from the eight-item PROMIS Anxiety Short Form Version 1.0 (National Institute of Neurological Disorders and Stroke 2015) along with the transformed *t*-score in the data bank. Note that the raw summed total score is labeled "Pre.Anx.sum," whereas the corresponding *t*-score is labeled "Pre.AnxT."

In this illustration, having the *t*-score table available will aid in identifying which *t*-score is assigned to the summated raw score. Table 8–2 offers published *t*-scores for the PROMIS Anxiety Short-Form Version 1.2. In this example, we must look up our mock sample patients' raw scores in the "Raw

	A	B	C	D	E	F	G	H	I	J	K	L	M	N
	First name	Last name	Med rec #	Pre. date	Pre. Anx1	Pre. Anx2	Pre. Anx3	Pre. Anx4	Pre. Anx5	Pre. Anx6	Pre. Anx7	Pre. Anx8	Pre. Anx.sum	Pre. AnxT
	John	Smith	1234	15-Jan	5	5	4	4	5	4	2	2	31	64.2
	Jane	Doe	2345	19-Jan	4	5	5	5	5	4	5	2	35	67.8
	David	Johnes	3456	20-Jan	5	4	5	3	5	5	4	3	34	66.8

FIGURE 8–2. Data bank formatting to capture raw and *t*-score measurement-based care by patient over time.

Anx=anxiety; AnxT=anxiety *t*-score; Pre.=pre-treatment (intake); rec=record.

TABLE 8–2.　PROMIS Neuro-QOL Anxiety Short Form *t*-score

Raw score	*t*-Score	SE
8	36.4	5.2
9	42.1	2.9
10	44.3	2.4
11	45.9	2.1
12	47.3	2.0
13	48.4	1.9
14	49.5	1.9
15	50.5	1.8
16	51.4	1.8
17	52.3	1.8
18	53.3	1.8
19	54.2	1.8
20	55.0	1.8
21	55.9	1.8
22	56.8	1.8
23	57.6	1.8
24	58.4	1.8
25	59.3	1.8
26	60.1	1.8
27	60.9	1.8
28	61.8	1.8
29	62.6	1.7
30	63.4	1.7
31	64.2	1.7
32	65.1	1.8
33	65.9	1.8
34	66.8	1.8
35	67.8	1.9
36	68.9	2.0
37	70.0	2.1
38	71.5	2.3
39	73.3	2.7
40	76.8	3.8

QOL=quality of life; SE=standard error.

score" column in the table to find their corresponding t-scores of 62.6 and 65.9, respectively. Navigating this extra step is worth the effort because if a scale has corresponding t-scores, then these are the ones that will be used for later data analyses. Reading t-tables may be painstaking; however, the process can be supplanted by programming a look-up calculation into Excel that will read the summed score in one cell and return the corresponding t-score in another column cell (in this case, the adjacent column). This will entail initial setup time to create the t-score transformation table in Excel and program the look-up action. The extra effort up front, however, will save minutes—if not hours—down the line.

Although transformed t-scores will be used in analyses more often than summated raw scores, keeping raw summated scores as part of the data bank is critical for interpretation. For example, John Smith's PROMIS Anxiety summed score is 31, which means we can determine his general tendency in response to the PROMIS Anxiety items by averaging his overall score. In this case, his average anxiety score is 3.9, which may indicate that John's anxiety symptoms are nearly occurring "often." Referring to the t-scores distribution in Table 8–2, we look for the corresponding t-score for the PROMIS Anxiety Short-Form Version 1.2 summary score of 31, which is 64.2. This indicates that John's reported anxiety is a little more than 1 standard deviation above the general population for anxiety. Armed with both data points provides a richer understanding of John's reported anxiety.

Cleaning Data

Once a data bank has been compiled, one is often eager to begin exploring. Before doing any basic pivot-table analyses or tossing the data into a statistical software, however, a thorough review to ensure the integrity of the data is necessary. Why? Because missing or erroneous data, such as data entry error or extreme outliers, can seriously draw into question the reliability and validity of MBC outcomes and skew the results (Cole 2008). Data cleaning is a critical part of data management to prepare a final product of high quality and thus *legitimacy*.

Proper data cleaning and subsequent editing should not be taken lightly. In the world of quantitative research, the vast mechanisms to clean and prepare data range from basic visual inspection and simple correction to complicated procedures such as bootstrapping to manage outliers or inverse probability weighting for missing data. If these latter procedures cause you to gasp for air, take heart that at this level of preparing aggregated MBC data, your focus only needs to be on simpler techniques to clean, edit, and ready your data. That said, should your data grow into larger sample sizes and have future use—for instance, for publication in a peer-reviewed journal article—you will want to employ a qualified data scientist to explore which of the vastly more advanced data cleaning methods are appropriate for your aggregated sample. For now, breathe a sigh of relief.

Many of the publications on proper data cleaning and editing techniques focus on big data sets and complicated studies that incorporate data mining from biomedical, neuropsychological, and epidemiological sources. Although preparing and cleaning MBC data may remain at the level of in-house QA or outreach dissemination, taking direction from this literature to guide data policy and procedures is always prudent. Even so, the manner in which MBC data are collected is a self-correcting process, thus reducing overreliance on many data cleaning guidelines. Because MBC data acquisition is conducted on a case-by-case basis between practitioner and patient, practitioners exercise notable control over naturally occurring data error simply by reviewing patient responses along the course of therapy. In other words, MBC data can be cleaned *in the course of data acquisition*. If missing data or patient errors are made, these can be corrected at the time of the therapeutic encounter before they are ever entered into the data bank. Adopting a mindset that data "cleaning" processes happen throughout MBC will reduce costs associated with staff time and loss of data. One method to ensure data accuracy is to do a quick scan to identify any missing or erroneous data on completion of the scales, while your patient is still present. If you find any irregularities, ask your patient to clarify them. Most errors and missing items can be caught at this point in the process.

If patients' data are wholly maintained, what remains as data management errors will most likely be due to 1) data entry error or 2) oversights in data-management processes. The former can be rectified by offering patients digitized questionnaires (removing staff data entry altogether) or requiring 100% double data-entry procedures to flag for keying errors if data entry is required. Any data-management errors can be moderated by appointing a data coordinator to manage and prepare MBC data following strict data management guidelines. The subsections that follow focus on basic considerations and approaches for cleaning data relevant to expected issues that may present while building an MBC data bank. We encourage you to explore weightier data cleaning solutions as your MBC program advances in size and complexity.

Missing Data

When patients intentionally or unintentionally leave values blank in a questionnaire, these are referred to as "missing data" and are a well-known problem most researchers face. Despite clinician control to review patient surveys as part of MBC (and thus address missing data), it would be naïve to expect that all data gathered by self-report will be 100% complete. Missing data may occur for various reasons. Patients might overlook and miss items on a survey or intentionally let certain questions go unanswered that they interpret as too sensitive, thus exercising their right not to answer such questions (McNeeley 2012). When exploring missing data, it is important to determine whether the absence of the data is due to arbitrary or random influences or to purposeful intent.

The data management literature refers to three types of missing data (Little et al. 2014; Rubin et al. 2007): 1) missing completely at random (MCAR), which means a response to a question was missed for no other reason than random oversight, 2) missing at random (MAR), which results in a sort of nuanced randomness in responding to an item (e.g., a question is not answered due to the effect from another survey question); or 3) missing not at random (MNAR), which means that a response to a question was purposefully left blank (e.g., refusal to answer sensitive questions). MCAR and MAR are very confusing to differentiate, we know. For the purposes of cleaning MBC data and to stay out of the weeds of nuance, we suggest simplifying "missingness" as a dichotomy of 1) random missing data and 2) intentional missing data. Determining whether data are missing intentionally or accidentally matters because of how it impacts data analysis and subsequent interpretation. For instance, random missing data can be addressed in ways to make the data set complete, whereas intentional missing data may present emerging patterns of missingness among a certain cohort of patients. Missingness in this latter instance is essentially *informative* and therefore must be interpreted and analyzed accordingly.

In building an MBC data bank, the data also should comprise demographic and psychiatric data, most often pulled from intake forms and medical records. Per Van den Broeck et al. (2005), missing data must be obtained and cleaned at all costs, including variables such as 1) gender (or biological sex), 2) gender identity specification, 3) age or birth date, and 4) testing date(s). This latter variable is of utmost importance to maintain the temporal integrity of the repeated-measures designs that are the methodological backbone of MBC. Demographic data can easily go missing during the process of transferring individual data into the MBC aggregated data bank, but this should not pose too difficult a task to fix. One can retrieve data by actively reviewing the medical record, directly asking the patient, or reviewing the hard copy questionnaires (if used) for missing data or dates. The inherent case-by-case review process of MBC reduces the likelihood of missing data, compared with the typical behavioral research study. Nevertheless, clinicians may still fail to see the missing data due to natural human oversight. If missing data are not dealt with correctly, especially those from scales aimed to determine cognitive, affective, and behavioral qualities, these missing values can nega-

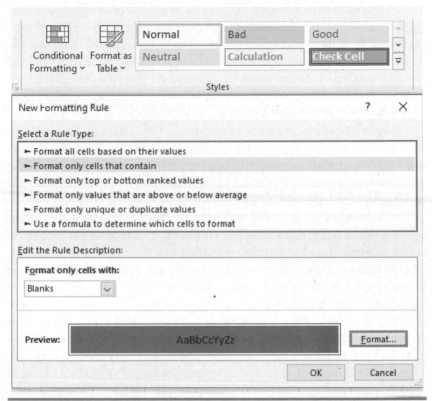

FIGURE 8–3. Microsoft Excel's point and click conditional formatting for identifying blank cells.
To view this figure in color, see Plate 4 in Color Gallery.

tively affect the validity and reliability of the summed scores when analyzed in group format (Çokluk and Kayri 2011).

There are simple ways to assess for missing items. If using an open-source spreadsheet such as Excel, simply sorting the data in ascending order will produce rows of blank cells at the top of the sort. Two other functions are available without disturbing the data set, but they require subsequent visual scanning to identify the patient for whom the data are missing. The first is to create a formula in each column at the bottom of the dataset to calculate the number of blank cells in that column (the "=countblank()" function). Newer versions of Microsoft Excel offer conditional formatting that, after a little reconnoitering, can be easily programmed to highlight blank cells using color. See Figure 8–3.

Once test variables are identified as missing, you must do something about it. Techniques for managing missing data are plentiful and can be found in a literature that has grown exponentially over the past decade. Garson (2015) noted that there is no simple rule to address missing values. Some approaches are simple procedures through basic calculations, whereas others require specialized simulation software attached to statistical data bases to fix the issue. According to Van den Broeck et al. (2005), approaches to correct missing data can be categorized in three ways: 1) ignore them, 2) change them, or 3) delete them. With the multiple tomes now dedicated to addressing missing data, it is easy for anyone to go down the data-editing rabbit hole. For purposes of managing a clinically driven MBC program, however, the best approach to correcting missing data will most likely be the simplest solution—of course, with the mindful caveat to choose "simple" when simple is the most appropriate and legitimate choice. Retracing steps back into the patient file to obtain the missing information is the simplest of all solutions to retrieve missing data, but two additional methods warrant further discussion.

One of the older, more traditional methods for addressing missing data (and the default in many statistical packages) was simply to throw them out. Choosing either listwise deletion (deleting the entire participant stream of data) or pairwise deletion (only tossing out those full measures with the missing values) can be detrimental to final analyses because it reduces the sample size (and therefore "power") and biasing estimates, which ultimately leads to limited generalization of findings (Cole 2008; Kang 2013; Schafer and Graham 2002). Removing a particular subset of patient data increases the risk of losing meaningful therapeutic outcomes associated with that cohort. If MNAR patterns (i.e., intentional missing data) for a particular group were overlooked and then deleted, what vital information was lost to the story of your treatment's impact with this cohort? Most opinions today are to avoid deleting cases altogether and to substitute missing data with estimated values (Piriyakul 2006; Rubin et al. 2007).

Nevertheless, circumstances exist in which dropping a case is warranted, especially with repeated measures designs such as MBC. For those patients who repeatedly produce incomplete surveys or consistently miss scheduled testing administrations, using their data after attempting to fix them through data editing may result in an inaccurate and artificial reflection of therapeutic progress. Thus, case deletion—in this regard—might be advisable and less disruptive. General guidelines suggest that when a few participants with missing data represent a small percentage of the overall sample and the data truly appear to be MAR, listwise deletion may be your best option (Osbourne 2013).

Another method to address missing data is to substitute them with an estimate. The simplest imputation method used for decades has been to employ "mean substitution," which takes two basic forms: person mean substitution (PMS) and item mean substitution (IMS). Although most researchers eschew single imputation mean substitution techniques for missing data, PMS continues to have credibility when items are missing from a psychological scale, such as those used in MBC. The notion is that it is more desirable to substitute patients' average mean score for the missing item than to discard their data altogether. PMS draws loosely on the psychological tenet that the best predictor of future behavior is past behavior; therefore, why not use one's existing scoring tendency as a substitute for one missing item? Downey and King (1998) further argued that because survey items are developed to correlate or hang with each other, and thus contribute to a calculated score of all other items in the scale, using PMS is an acceptable solution.

PMS is calculated by averaging the answered items left in the symptom scale for which the missing value is identified, then substituting that averaged value into the missing value. John Smith's PHQ-9 data illustrate this. In Figure 8–4, the datum was missing for PHQ-9 item 4 (which, hypothetically, was alerted by the conditional formatting program to change the empty cell's color). Averaging the eight available data yielded the mean substitution score of 2.375 shown in that cell. Note that the substituted score inflated John Smith's original summed score found in Figure 8–1 by 0.375. In the absence of any other information, the mean is the best single estimate of one's score (Parent 2013).

IMS is also based on averaging the scores of a psychological test, but across all participants in the sample. IMS calculates the average of the variable from other individuals in the sample who reported data for that item. The average of that item is then substituted into the missing value. In other cases, the IMS comprises the overall aggregate sample mean of a scale, which is then substituted for missing items within that scale. It is assumed that the mean is an assumed single value of what would have been observed if that item were completed (Little et al. 2014). What appears as a simple solution to randomly missing item data becomes a little more complicated when composite or subscales comprise a psychological test. In these instances, either PMS or IMS must be calculated using only those subscale items. Osbourne (2013) advised that when a symptom scale's internal consistency is strong, occasional use of mean substitution is not likely to affect the overall covariance of the scale (Schafer and Graham 2002).

The limitations of using single imputation mean substitution is that, despite preserving the mean score for a particular scale in the sample, the very act of substituting an average score to replace a raw data point reduces the natural variance of the sample distribution. Should a patient's symptom scale be missing more than 20% of the data, mean substitution would likely "over fit" the data, yielding a reduced capacity to generalize findings (Osbourne 2013). Additionally, as the number of mean substitution events increases, these corrections will inflate the distribution of the data toward artificial homogeneity, thereby negatively impacting parametric analyses. The rule

	A	B	C	D	E	F	G	H	I	J	K	L	M	N
	First name	Last name	Med rec #	Pre. date	Pre. PHQ1	Pre. PHQ2	Pre. PHQ3	Pre. PHQ4	Pre. PHQ5	Pre. PHQ6	Pre. PHQ7	Pre. PHQ8	Pre. PHQ9	Pre. PHQ.sum
2	John	Smith	1234	15-Jan	3	3	2	2.375	1	3	3	1	3	21.375
3	Jane	Doe	2345	19-Jan	2	2	3	3	3	3	2	2	3	23
4	David	Johnes	3456	20-Jan	3	2	3	3	2	1	1	3	2	20

FIGURE 8–4. Example of person mean substitution method using Microsoft Excel.

PHQ=Patient Health Questionnaire; Pre.=pre-treatment (intake); rec=record.

TABLE 8–3. Percentage of missing data items allowed per symptom scale total items

Total number of scale items	Missing scale items allowed				
	1%	5%	10%	15%	20%
5 questions	0.05	0.25	0.50	0.75	1.00
7 questions	0.07	0.35	0.70	1.05	1.40
10 questions	0.10	0.50	1.00	1.50	2.00
15 questions	0.15	0.75	1.50	2.25	3.00
20 questions	0.20	1.00	2.00	3.00	4.00
25 questions	0.25	1.25	2.50	3.75	5.00
30 questions	0.30	1.50	3.00	4.50	6.00

of thumb is to use single imputation mean substitution only when <20% of the scale items are missing (Downey and King 1998; Osbourne 2013; Parent 2013; Piriyakul 2006) and when 1%–5% of other data are missing (e.g., single scores, demographics) (Little et al. 2014; Piriyakul 2006; Rubin et al. 2007). Table 8–3 provides a guideline of percentage estimates of how many missing item values are allowed based on the total number of total scale items.

Other robust estimation substitution methods are available that are arguably more rigorous, with fewer disadvantageous effects on a data sample, including regression, hot deck, maximum likelihood, and multiple imputations. Elaborating on these is outside the scope of this book because these methods are preferred for big data studies, which may not be applicable to an emerging MBC program. We encourage you to investigate missing data correction methods as your MBC data sets continue to grow and expand. Handbooks well worth the investment on the subject include

- Enders C: *Applied Missing Data Analysis*. New York, Guilford, 2010
- Little RJA, Rubin DB: *Statistical Analysis With Missing Data*. Hoboken, NJ, Wiley, 2002
- Osbourne JW: *Best Practices in Data Cleaning: A Complete Guide to Everything You Need to Do Before and After Collecting Your Data*. Thousand Oaks, CA, Sage, 2013

Outliers and Erroneous Data

When scanning your data set for missing data through the sorting method described earlier, you may come upon extreme scores that you would not have expected for a particular variable. When a data point differs significantly from other observations, or if the data values are inconsistent with other values in the distribution (Zimek and Filzmoser 2018), then you likely have what is known as an "outlier" (less commonly referred to as "influential data points") (Osbourne 2013). The deviation of the value in outliers, whether they are extremely small or extremely large, can be problematic on many fronts. If these values are not identified and edited, they may distort the data interpretation because outliers may not be a genuine reflection of the participant's input (Cousineau and Chartier 2010). They also can cause serious problems in statistical analyses, especially parametric statistics in which the assumptions of normal distribution and calculation of the arithmetic mean are violated.

Like missing data, it is essential to determine how outliers occur and whether they are simply erroneous data or have occurred organically within your sample. The latter, once identified, are no longer "outliers" but "novelties" (Santoyo 2017). In most cases, however, the error occurred during data collection, entry, or management, and any extreme scores recorded from the symptom scales collected for MBC will most likely be erroneous. However, depending on the clinic or facility, some of the data you are interested in incorporating into MBC might be biomedical (i.e., blood pressure) or pharmaceutical (i.e., medication dosage). If outliers from these sources are discovered, it is important to double-check for equipment failure or recorded inaccuracies. If outliers are found to be erroneous, the most logical fix is to go back to the original record and reenter the correct value or to remeasure the patient if that is feasible and appropriate. If neither option is possible, many researchers recommend removing the data altogether (Rousseeuw and Hubert 2018) or replacing the value as you would for missing data (Van den Broeck et al. 2005). Whatever method you choose, it is imperative to document these occurrences and the procedures used to fix them.

When the extreme value is a legitimate data point—a novelty—then it is advisable to leave it as it is. An outlier skewing the aggregated findings is not enough reason to drop that data point. In fact, dropping the case with the outlier will artificially "normalize" your data and increase Type I errors (assuming meaningful significance when there is none). It is bad practice to remove data points to yield a better-fitting model (Frost 2019). For example, imagine a scenario that is not too terribly "outlier-ish" but rather is likely to occur in clinical practice: during data cleaning, you observe that most of your patients' ages range between 35 and 55 years old, but further inspection reveals two patients with ages that fall on either end of the distribution, say, a patient who is 22 years old and another who is 75. Do you drop these cases when studying the effects of your treatment? Tightening up the data by removing outliers limits opportunities to learn about the reach of your treatment program. In this example, retaining all of the cases allows for deeper exploration by studying whether your therapy has had a therapeutic impact based on age distribution. A good data analyst or statistician slated to analyze your sample will understand how to organize these scores and determine the extent to which variation has contributed to your outcomes.

We highly recommend establishing predetermined rules to manage any missing or outlying data. Along with a data dictionary, you should also have a set of guidelines for cleaning your data. Each instance of data editing is imperative to document. When it comes to final reporting, noting the number of missing values, data errors, and outliers in the your data set, along with the steps you took to correct them, will ensure the legitimacy of your aggregated sample.

Securing Data

Whether you hire an outside firm to manage your MBC data or develop your own program in-house, taking the steps to ensure patient data remain secure is vital to the overall success of MBC. If hiring an outside commercial service is the objective, then thoroughly understanding how that company plans to maintain data security and give you access to it will be essential for peace of mind and patient privacy rights.

According to William Michener (2015), a common assumption that researchers make is that their personal computers live forever. A good data management plan should include procedures for routinely duplicating data files and archiving data banks into secure locations, such as an external hard drive or a company shared drive. The plan should include making scheduled backups and ensuring that stored data files can be retrieved. If you are part of a larger facility that employs an information technology team, we recommend working with these colleagues to routinely secure and encrypt MBC data. In some cases, remote storage locations may be viable for keeping extra copies of your data set. Some commercial internet services, such as Dropbox or Google, can serve as off-site storage, but you must ensure that wherever you store your data meets the criteria for HIPAA compliance. Nostalgically speaking, nothing is more secure than a locked file cabinet in a locked office.

Once the data have been aggregated and are ready for analysis, patient information should be deidentified as part of the security backup and storage plan. Two sets of files, hard copy and electronic, that are kept under separate lock and key should contain patients' names as they are assigned to the deidentified code. These stringent security steps also apply to how MBC hard files are stored. Whether you are in an independent private practice or a member of a larger facility, the care given to patient files is the same care needed to secure the MBC portfolio of questionnaires, graphs, and qualitative reports.

Data Analysis

The objective of this section is not to subjugate you, dear reader, with a crash course in basic and intermediate statistics but simply to outline two data analytic methods for organizing and presenting MBC data. The first approach covers how basic statistics can be run through an open-source spreadsheet, such as Excel, for the purpose of QA review or general outreach dissemination. The second approach offers an outline of applicable statistical methods for which an MBC data set is most suited. As your facility's MBC data bank continues to grow, eventually these data will be large enough for inferential statistical analyses either to determine the extent of change or to assess the correlates of therapeutic change, ultimately producing the story of your patients' overall treatment progress and your therapeutic program's effectiveness. When you get to this point, it is may be advisable to call in that old favor from an academic peer or to hire a behavioral science statistician.

Unless you have achieved the requisite skill set or training to conduct statistical methods, you should be cautious when preparing MBC data into aggregate form and "analyzing" the findings. Employing proper statistical analysis is fundamental to ethically reporting data; any misuse—whether intentional or accidental—is a great disservice to both the scientific community and the public at large (Nelson et al. 2000). We encourage you, therefore, to implement the procedures outlined in this section and ask that you incorporate these methods within your scope of practice and confidence. Responsible use of assessment data is bound by the rigors of the American Statistical Association (2018), which expects us to approach data in a professional, competent, respectful, and ethical manner.

Statistics to Describe MBC

Once the MBC data are organized, cleaned, properly stored, and safely contained in a spreadsheet, running basic descriptive statistics will be the next step. The data do not necessarily have to be transferred to a statistical software to run basic descriptive statistics; Microsoft Excel and LibreOffice Calc offer these calculations as part of their suites. Nevertheless, without some spreadsheet proficiency, you are likely better off transferring your data to a statistical program that will analyze them from simple (descriptive) to advanced (inferential) statistics.

A data sample is described by running it through descriptive statistics. These calculations are the method by which data are organized and summarized, yielding insight and trends of a sample. The resulting analyses do not draw conclusions about your patients; they *describe* the sample (hence the name), summarizing how the data group together and how they vary. In

MBC, this could be an overview of who your patients are and how they self-reported their therapeutic progress. Another benefit of descriptive statistics is to use them to double-check for outliers and missing or erroneous values. Frequency distributions of descriptive statistics (i.e., how many times did a certain value occur?) will show the number of missing and extreme values for any variable. Running descriptive statistics is usually the first step in data analysis because they help identify errors and create the backdrop for the data to tell the story of your MBC process. Themes emerge when descriptive statistics are run; for instance, questions such as the typical age range, gender distribution, presenting conditions, symptom severity, and even the average degree of reported change of your sample can be gleaned from this process.

For researchers, conducting descriptive statistics is typically the first step before running the data through hypothesis testing by means of more advanced, inferential analyses. For the MBC practitioner, running descriptive statistics conceivably could be both your first and last step if the data are not used beyond QA purposes. This is fine. The aim of MBC is to augment the clinical process, not to conduct research on patients. Using descriptive statistics to create graphic illustrations of your data (e.g., bar charts and line graphs) for in-house purposes, such as QA, clinical staff education, or leadership reporting, can demonstrate your patients' therapeutic progress more than using tables of central tendency, range, and dispersion. Figure 8–5 shows how descriptive statistics (the mock PHQ-9 data initially presented in Figure 8–1) can be recorded in Excel and subsequently produce a line graph of the aggregated sample's average reported depression symptoms over time. Both the tables and the graph use the same data to convey therapeutic change over time. Due to the small sample size, some measures of central tendency (i.e., "mode") and the shape of the distribution of scores (i.e., "kurtosis") will show error output.

Statistics to Estimate Change

In Part II we outlined how MBC methods are akin to the single-subject design evidence-based practice research. Using the single-subject approach is a sound method for collecting progress data over the course of psychotherapy (i.e., MBC), and when patients are aggregated together to compose a collective sample, this continuance lends itself to be examined as a within-subjects, repeated-measures longitudinal study (i.e., outcomes research). Analyzing data through repeated-measures approaches means repeatedly measuring the same outcome variable on the same individual over time to determine whether the extent of progress or change is statistically significant.

At the individual level, the reliable change index (RCI) was introduced to assess the likelihood of therapeutic change by controlling for test error variance. At the aggregated sample level, RCI is still a viable and accepted

Pre.PHQ.sum		Wk2.PHQ.sum		Wk4.PHQ.sum	
Mean	21.3	Mean	19.0	Mean	12.3
Standard error	0.882	Standard error	0.577	Standard error	2.333
Median	21.0	Median	19.0	Median	13.0
Mode	#N/A	Mode	#N/A	Mode	#N/A
Standard deviation	1.528	Standard deviation	1.000	Standard deviation	4.041
Sample variance	2.333	Sample variance	1.000	Sample variance	16.333
Kurtosis	#DIV/0!	Kurtosis	#DIV/0!	Kurtosis	#DIV/0!
Skewness	0.9	Skewness	0.0	Skewness	-0.7
Range	3	Range	2	Range	8
Minimum	20	Minimum	18	Minimum	8
Maximum	23	Maximum	20	Maximum	16
Sum	64	Sum	57	Sum	37
Count	3	Count	3	Count	3

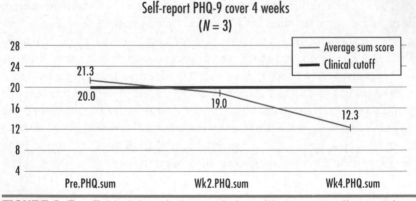

FIGURE 8–5. Tabled descriptive statistics with summary line-graph averages plotted over time using a Microsoft Excel spreadsheet.

PHQ=Patient Health Questionnaire; Pre.=pre-treatment (intake); rec=record; Wk=week.

measure to assess change; in fact, others have reported that RCI can yield findings that are as accurate and consistent regarding change over time as its more complex (and complicated) statistical comrades, such as regression analysis (Heaton et al. 2001). The purpose of this section is to outline the usefulness of other change statistics once your data sample is large enough to meet the power requirements for more advanced statistics, such as Cohen's *d*, repeated-measures analysis of variance (ANOVA), and various regressions methods. Each analytic approach is introduced with the intent to bolster your general understanding when considering analyzing MBC outcomes and to pique your curiosity for further reading.

Effect Size

Effect size is a statistic that shows the standardized difference between two mean scores with respect to the magnitude of change, often assumed to be due to an intervention. The effect size calculus can be used to determine the size of the difference between two means in two distinct groups or to determine the size of an effect within the same group when measured at different times, such as in MBC (i.e., how *big* is the difference between reported pre-treatment functioning and post-treatment functioning?). Effect size calculations are especially important to evidenced-based treatment outcomes and, therefore, to MBC.

Most readers will be familiar with the effect size calculation of Cohen's *d* (Cohen 1988) yet perhaps less familiar with another calculation, Hedges' *g*, which is just as valuable, especially with smaller sample sizes (Hedges and Olkin 1985). Both estimations calculate effect size by taking the difference of two means and dividing it by the pooled standard deviation (Cohen's *d*) or by the weighted standard deviation (Hedges' *g*). It has been argued that Hedges' *g* provides a more "corrected" version to the biased estimate of Cohen's *d* (Lakens 2013). Other effect size calculations, eta squared (or "η^2") and partial-eta squared, are included in the output of inferential statistics, such as ANOVA and regression, as indices of the proportion of variance based on observed effects (Richardson 2011). The magnitude of *d* and *g* effect sizes are interpreted using Cohen's (1988) guideline to consider the size of change ranging typically from small (0.20) to large (0.80), and for η^2, these range from small (0.06) to large (0.14).

Repeated Measures Analysis of Variance

To compare whether the mean scores between two separate groups are significantly different, it is typical to run an independent samples *t*-test. When there are more than two groups to compare, the statistic used to compare means then becomes the ANOVA. To compare mean scores from the same group of people taken at two different times, say at pre-treatment and then at post-treatment, a paired samples *t*-test is used. As we add more intervals of measurement to determine change over time, like with MBC, the repeated measures ANOVA (RM-ANOVA) is employed; this is often considered an extension of the paired samples *t*-test (Sullivan 2008) and is suitable for MBC, especially when the sample size is estimated to be large enough for statistical power.

One of the defining features of the RM-ANOVA for within-subjects analyses is that it accounts for the variance that hypothetically occurs between assessments for each participant; this assumes that when data are repeatedly collected for an individual they will be more *similar* than data collected repeatedly from different groups (Koh and Sadigov 2010). Therefore, the collection of repeated data is correlative or "dependent." The RM-ANOVA takes the ratio of the sample variance (due to treatment effects) in relation to the error variance to determine change over time (Sullivan 2008). In this sense, it considers each patient as their own control when analyzing change over time (Singh et al. 2013). Like most parametric statistics, certain assumptions must be met before conducting RM-ANOVA, the most important being sphericity. This assumption requires that the variances of each time interval assessment be the same.

Regression

Beyond RM-ANOVA are several other advanced statistical models for assessing change. One of these is in the family of ANOVAs; the multivariate analysis of variance (MANOVA) is an extension of the ANOVA when there are two or more dependent (outcome) variables, and it examines the covariance of outcome variables to compare sample means. Another set of parametric statistics that is frequently used to understand repeated measures data are those in the regression-based approaches to evaluate change. These include ordinary least squares regression, ordinal logistic regression, hierarchical regression, and hierarchical linear modeling, just to name a few (because there are many). Regression methods are some of the more popular approaches for predicting behavior or forecasting the market, understanding the extent of influence among variables, determining the strength of the relationship between variables, and establishing the degree of change over time. It is this latter purpose that we briefly address.

Regression analyses are essentially about determining the relationship between two or more variables, sort of like correlations on steroids. Regressions often are referred to as "equations" because of the stepped nature in placing independent, dependent, and confounding variables to build the statistical model. Generally speaking, the goal of regression is to estimate how changes in the independent variable(s) relate to changes in the outcomes variable by holding constant or "controlling" for every variable included into the equation. This allows us to explain the effects of change that one variable has on another without having to worry about the effects of any other confounds. This comes in handy when wishing to understand aggregated MBC data due to the observational or naturalistic nature in which we collect this information. Regression takes into account the variability in patient responses and assumes that that same patient variability will be accounted for throughout data acquisition.

MBC data from two time points, say, pre- and post-treatment, will serve as the independent (predictor) variable and the dependent (outcome) variable, respectively, in the regression equation. By holding the independent variable "constant" (in addition to any confounding variables we add, such as age, sex, socioeconomic status), the regression will indicate the degree of association between the baseline value and outcome and account for any initial between-group differences when establishing whether any observed pre- to post-treatment differences are due to the treatment itself, differences in the groups at baseline, or a combination of these factors.

As we mentioned, there are many regression equations from which to choose, and an important deciding factor is whether the regression model you have chosen fits the nature of your data. For example, we discussed nominal, ordinal, interval, and ratio data earlier, and there is a regression equation to manage all of these data classifications. When the MBC data are Likert-type scaled data or ordinal data, choosing an ordinal linear regression may be appropriate. The most common choice for the linear regression, however, is the ordinary least squares regression, which requires continuous scaled data (interval and ratio scales). As with all inferential statistics, certain assumptions must be met to run your data through regression. First, the relationship between the dependent and independent variables is assumed to be linear, which would likely be the case with MBC data because each variable is produced by the same participant over time. Other assumptions have to do with the manner in which the data points "scatter" or fit the predictive regression line. These distances are called "residuals" and must meet the assumption of independence and have constant variance across all levels.

As MBC advances beyond the individual aspect to promote treatment success and into larger platforms of aggregated patient data, progressive forms of regression methods, for example, structural equation modeling, will likely be the statistical method of choice. In these scenarios, multiple practice variables can be entered into the "equation" to assess the extent to which they contribute to the outcomes of psychotherapy or psychiatric care. These include deeper dives into factors associated with comorbidity, effects of polypharmacy, and integrative treatment approaches. By integrating MBC into our clinical practices, we are inherently launching the behavioral health industry as a whole to new heights of multifaceted approaches to ensure treatment success, which will promote new research agendas to study and thus a practice-based evidence paradigm.

PART V

Moving Beyond Simple Progress Monitoring

*Implications for Practitioners and
a New Practice Paradigm*

From Personalized Patient-Centered Care to Practice-Based Evidence

As noble souls who have chosen a career in the mental health healing profession, our education exposed us to many varying orientations from which we developed our therapeutic style, treatment preferences, and allegiance to schools of thought or practice. We do what we do because we want to help others get better, get sober, reduce suffering, and so on. There are many more lucrative careers out there besides working in the behavioral health care industry. Our "success" in this field has more to do with helping others obtain recovery than with earning big, fat paychecks. Therefore, the manner in which we practice our approaches to help heal carries great weight and meaning. Successful therapeutic outcomes are not only our goal but also a direct measure of how effective our treatment efforts are.

Patient testimonial most often is our measure of success. This form of feedback bolsters our clinical confidence, strengthens our convictions, and, for some of us, warms our hearts. Yet as we traverse the landscape of managed care and the ever-advancing world of accreditation agencies, the "warm fuzzies" of testimony will not entirely sustain us. Measurement-based care (MBC) can bridge this gap. We have discussed how the primary function of MBC, at the individual level, is to improve patient treatment outcomes, support patient-centered care, and enhance clinical practice. Allow us now to briefly consider how—in aggregate form—it will serve to uphold your own clinical practice standards. Exploring the systemic benefits of implementing an MBC infrastructure will likewise satisfy the requirements of accreditation and embolden your affiliation with managed care.

The Clinician: How MBC Feedback Loops Feed Back to Clinicians

In our clinical experience, we explain therapeutic progress data to patients via easy-to-read colorful graphs of their psychological profile. These handouts have become exceedingly popular and are seen by patients and clinical staff alike as "therapeutic report cards." There appears to be a validating effect for both clinician and patient when verbal, qualitative experiential reports are combined with quantitative data. Furthermore, an additional and unexpected benefit we have seen—and one not yet discussed in the literature—has been how MBC strengthens the relationships among members of the clinical treatment team. The opportunity that MBC offers the clinician has evinced deeper collaboration and appreciation among interdisciplinary colleagues. The following is feedback from a clinician who is a member of an interdisciplinary team:

> The collaboration of the team is one of my favorite parts of measurement-based care. Patients feel like they are getting great care because it was very clear the treatment team was communicating and invested in them. They really appreciated seeing their data progress, as well as hearing about their progress. The data from progress evaluations also allowed us to collaborate on reiterating the importance of continuing care; in fact, some of my patients changed their mind and agreed to sober-living/[partial hospitalization] based on the meeting. The process also helped me to hear the medical provider's perspective too, to see his relationship with patients, which allowed me to observe patients in a different way. This gave me some insight into what treatment goals needed to be adjusted. Treatment goals were often adjusted, which was a direct result of seeing the data midway through.

MBC has shown us that the sweetness of therapeutic alliance goes both ways, as well as bringing clinician teams closer together, with greater appreciation for each other. On more than one occasion we have heard clinicians express how the process of MBC reminded them of why they do what they do in the first place. Might these feedback loops on feedback help reduce caregiver burnout or lead to more job satisfaction? Could such tertiary gains contribute to better treatment outcomes because of the additional support that MBC provides to clinicians? Goodman et al. (2013) outlined how MBC could benefit novice clinicians by substantiating their clinical skills, but we have seen directly how this process also has encouraged our seasoned veterans. Who doesn't like a little validation here and there?

To move beyond the primary function at the individual level, the method in which MBC data are compiled must also incorporate strategies so that individual data are captured and grouped together, or "aggregated." When combining your cases in this manner and reviewing therapeutic progress change in aggregate form, you are essentially producing your own programmatic report card. Depending on the number of psychometric scales administered, the combinations in analyses can yield a multitude of varying angles. For instance, the data can be sorted by which patients received a particular therapeutic approach, by age, by primary diagnosis, by length of treatment, or a combination of demographics. It is not necessary to dive into advanced statistical analyses by any means; what is necessary is that practitioners be able to observe their aggregated patient data in such a way that they may understand trends in treatment effectiveness. This represents one of the differences between clinical and statistical significance. This also becomes the feedback loop on which we gauge treatment outcomes. Questions about treatment effectiveness or program fidelity can be answered by progress data such as

- To what extent did my patients improve (or report symptom reduction)?
- What is the average length of time in therapy that reported changes begin to occur?
- Do the data align well with my clinical judgment?
- What are the trends in overall patient progress?

For managers, these types of questions may entail identifying which of your clinical staff are better at working with a given population over another. Obtaining trended information to answer such treatment-effectiveness questions can not only maintain best practices but, when appropriate, be used for marketing outreach efforts (albeit ensuring those claims are consistent with statistical principles). Additionally, these are the types of questions that accrediting agencies such as The Joint Commission and third-party payers wish to review. The reach of MBC is considerable. What initially was purported to enhance behavioral health care at the individual level is now at the heart of the practice-based evidence movement (Ammerman et al. 2014).

The Practice: How MBC Heightens Personalized Medicine

The new century began with a successful shift away from the paternalistic medical model to patient-centered care and soon after to personalized medicine. These now-popular practice modalities represent the bandwagon to which most of us aspire or on which we already ride. Practicing psychotherapy, psychiatric medicine, or medicine in general that emphasizes patient-focused and -tailored, personalized approaches, is a marked improvement from and all-around better clinical care than paternalistic medicine. Paternalistic medicine represented a clear delineation of top-down delivery of information, expecting the practitioner to be expert advisor and director of treatment decision-making and the patient to be the compliant recipient of treatment. Patient-centered care shifted the power in the doctor–patient relationship to become collaborative, and with it came shared treatment decision-making (Taylor 2009). Furthermore, practitioners are now expected to learn more about patient values, needs, and quality of life as critical pieces of overall treatment approaches (Gask and Coventry 2012).

It is arguable that the practice of psychiatry and psychotherapy has always emphasized a patient-centered approach, with its emphasis on the doctor–patient (or clinician–client) relationship, collaborative care, and art of "active listening," But patient-centered care is more than this; it is also more than simply placing the patient in the "center" of treatment focus. The Institute of Medicine (2001) defined patient-centered care as "care that is respectful of and responsive to individual patient preferences, needs, and values and ensures that patient values guide all clinical decisions" (p. 6). Collaboration between provider and patient during treatment entails considering patients' overall quality of life at all times and their involvement in treatment decision-making, for which meaningful goals go beyond symptom reduction to include enhanced quality of life and better functioning (Dixon and Lieberman 2014). A secondary gain to patient-centered care is that it places greater responsibility on the patient, which may in turn likely improve treatment compliance. The nature of communication is clearly one of the main adaptations that occurred as a result of the shift from paternalistic to patient-centered care. In each of these instances, MBC plays a clinically meaningful role in augmenting the doctor–patient (clinician–client) relationship and communication.

In the current milieu of managed care, in-depth and lengthy conversations that align with patient-centered medicine to assess patient preferences, needs, and values may pose a logistical nightmare for some practices. Therefore, the inclusion of MBC may serve several additional functions to enhance the patient-centered care practice. The first of these is personalization; the well-chosen instrument(s), in terms of its relevance to your practice objectives, can summarize presenting problems, important beliefs and values, and the social determinants necessary for well-rounded conceptualization. The data gleaned from this process can yield important unique patient information that will further tailor treatment planning to meet that patient's distinct needs and desires. In essence, this embodies "personalized medicine" because the information gathered is used to determine the best treatment for each patient. The second and third functions are about time efficiency and its impact on doctor–patient communication. The time taken to administer psychometric evaluations will be markedly less than that needed to glean such information in a traditional clinical interview. Consequently, more time is made available in the therapy hour to *actually do* therapy and clinical work and to establish rapport and therapeutic alliance, and less time is needed for perfunctory "interviewing." Having more one-on-one time with your patient further supports the quality of patient-centered care.

Repeated use of psychometric measures to establish therapeutic progress enhances patient-centered care and personalized treatment because it is—quite simply—a repeated extension of the initial process to evaluate patient values, quality of life changes, symptom severity variations, and so on. With each review of therapeutic progress via MBC, you are essentially appraising and reappraising the integrity and applicability of your treatment approach and plan. Personalized treatment through MBC thus becomes a dynamic and engaging process.

The Field: Role of MBC in Practice-Based Evidence

In many ways, MBC represents the long-awaited marriage of science and practice. Despite their rocky courtship, exemplified by the smug view of researchers, who assume that what they produce the clinician will use, and by the perceived stubbornness of clinicians, who insist on conducting treatment as they see fit (Green 2008), a bridge to a new, integrated "best practice" is conceivably manifested through MBC. Integrating the element of quantifiable measures and its requisite methods into the clinical repertoire substantively transforms standard practice into MBC practice. Clinicians continue to be the driving force, conducting psychotherapeutic or psychiatric care as they see fit while employing tools of the evidence-based research trade to enhance therapeutic progress and substantiate clinical outcomes.

The reach of augmenting MBC into clinical practice has the potential to yield more than just the expected benefits to the individual in therapy; it may play an important role in elevating the behavioral health profession. In recent years, the impetus to expand the applicability of evidenced-based practices verified through randomized controlled trials (RCTs) continues to gain momentum. Burgeoning research agendas such as translational research (Woolf 2008; Zerhouni 2007), implementation science (Bauer and Kirchner 2020; Bauer et al. 2015; Perry et al. 2019), pragmatic research (Glasgow 2013; Holtrop and Glasgow 2020), and practice-based evidence (Green 2008; Lieberman et al. 2010; Swisher 2010) tend to share common concerns, such as 1) how do established evidence-based practices (EBPs) translate to serve various communities and 2) can the methods of EBP practice treatment delivery vary across given populations to reach the same clinical outcomes? These concerns are not new to practicing clinicians; our implementation of MBC essentially allows us to examine these objectives at the microcosmic level of clinical practice. When choosing an intervention to help a patient reach a desired outcome and to monitor their progress through MBC, we essentially substantiate whether that intervention was effective in achieving those outcomes. In this instance, you are basically conducting practice-based evidence.

What is clear at the time of this writing is that the field of mental health has entered a new paradigm. The vision of many thought leaders (discussed in and referenced throughout this book) has propelled our collective thinking to question the absolute authority of the over-controlled, sterilized environment of the RCT that produces the evidence-based treatments we use to conduct therapy. This is not to claim that such trials are no longer relevant (far from it) but to engender further consideration of studying the human condition through more realistic and, thus, more readily applicable approaches. Given that greater focus is placed on patient-centered care or personalized medicine, how might patients' values, cultural influences, needs, and quality-of-life functioning be considered measurable factors in RCTs and not just confounding variables that need to be controlled?

An example of thinking outside the RCT-EBP box relates to what was once another confound in evidence-based research, coined "non-specifics" of psychotherapy. For decades, clinician characteristics of therapeutic alliance, perceived competence, and relational components of therapy were considered confounds or "noise" in RCT studies (as have been *participant* factors such as race, socioeconomic status, and comorbidities). MBC research helped uncover (or perhaps rediscover) that such "confounding variables" actually mean a whole lot more to clinical outcomes than just a set of variables to "control" (Chatoor and Krupnick 2001). In fact, Miller et al. (2008) aptly noted that practicing clinicians have far greater influence on treatment outcomes than EBP alone. Devising methods to design EBP studies around the messy, variable nature of humanness is critical to the field of mental health, given that it is made up by two sets of messy variable humans: those who seek our help and those of us who provide it.

The MBC initiative dovetails beautifully with the practice-based evidence paradigm. As science has informed practice with respect to evidence-based treatment, so practice will inform science with respect to how well those EBP protocols are working in the community. MBC offers the methodology by which practice-based approaches can be utilized to further strengthen the noble work of mental health. What you do at the individual level with MBC to ensure your patient is making the most of psychotherapy, you also do to inform the greater collective.

Pun intended. The opportunities are immeasurable.

Appendix A: Why-What-How Operationalization Worksheet

My why: Professional mission statement

What I treat: Operationalizing conditions	
Condition	Measurable constructs

How I treat it: Operationalizing approaches	
Therapeutic method	Measurable constructs

Appendix B: Stakeholders Graphic

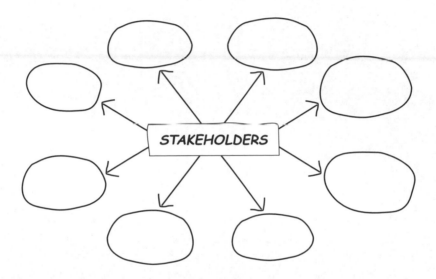

STAKEHOLDERS

References

Althubaiti A: Information bias in health research: definition, pitfalls, and adjustment methods. J Multidiscip Healthc 9:211–217, 2016 27217764

American Educational Research Association, American Psychological Association, National Council on Measurement in Education: Standards for Educational and Psychological Testing. Washington, DC, American Educational Research Association, 2014. Available at: www.testingstandards.net/uploads/7/6/6/4/76643089/standards_2014edition.pdf. Accessed January 12, 2022.

American Psychiatric Association: Diagnostic and Statistical Manual of Mental Disorders, 5th Edition. Arlington, VA, American Psychiatric Association, 2013

American Psychological Association: Ethical Principles of Psychologists and Code of Conduct. Washington, DC, American Psychological Association, 2010. Available at: www.apa.org/ethics/code. Accessed January 12, 2022.

American Statistical Association: Ethical Guidelines for Statistical Practice. Prepared by the Committee on Professional Ethics of the American Statistical Association. Alexandria, VA, American Statistical Association, April 14, 2018. Available at: www.amstat.org/asa/files/pdfs/EthicalGuidelines.pdf. Accessed January 12, 2022.

Ammerman A, Smith TW, Calancie L: Practice-based evidence in public health: improving reach, relevance, and results. Annu Rev Public Health 35:47–63, 2014 24641554

Anastasi A, Urbina S: Psychological Testing, 7th Edition. Upper Saddle River, NJ, Prentice-Hall, 1997

Ashford RD, Brown A, Brown T, et al: Defining and operationalizing the phenomena of recovery: a working definition from the recovery science research collaborative. Addict Res Theory 27(3):179–188, 2019

Bauer MS, Kirchner J: Implementation science: what is it and why should I care? Psychiatry Res 283:112376, 2020 31036287

Bauer MS, Damschroder L, Hagedorn H, et al: An introduction to implementation science for the non-specialist. BMC Psychol 3(1):32, 2015 26376626

Beck JS: Cognitive Behavior Therapy: Basics and Beyond, 2nd Edition. New York, Guilford, 2011

Beckstead DJ, Hatch AL, Lambert MJ, et al: Clinical significance of the Outcome Questionnaire (OQ-45.2). Behav Anal Today 4(1):86–97, 2003

Belk RA, Pilling M, Rogers KD, et al: The theoretical and practical determination of clinical cut-offs for the British Sign Language versions of PHQ-9 and GAD-7. BMC Psychiatry 16(1):372–384, 2016 27809821

Bickman L, Kelley SD, Breda C, et al: Effects of routine feedback to clinicians on mental health outcomes of youths: results of a randomized trial. Psychiatr Serv 62(12):1423–1429, 2011 22193788

Bischoff T, Anderson SR, Heafner J, et al: Establishment of a reliable change index for the GAD-7. Psychol Community Health 8(1):176–187, 2020

Boswell JF, Kraus DR, Castonguay LG, et al: Treatment outcome package: measuring and facilitating multidimensional change. Psychotherapy (Chic) 52(4):422–431, 2015 26641372

Byiers BJ, Reichle J, Symons FJ: Single-subject experimental design for evidence-based practice. Am J Speech Lang Pathol 21(4):397–414, 2012 23071200

Campbell DT, Fiske DW: Convergent and discriminant validation by the multi-trait-multimethod matrix. Psychol Bull 56(2):81–105, 1959 13634291

Carifio J, Perla RJ: Ten common misunderstandings, misconceptions, persistent myths and urban legends about Likert Scales and Likert Response Formats and their antidotes. J Soc Sci 3(3):106–116, 2007

Cella D, Riley W, Stone A, et al: The Patient-Reported Outcomes Measurement Information System (PROMIS) developed and tested its first wave of adult self-reported health outcome item banks: 2005–2008. J Clin Epidemiol 63(11):1179–1194, 2010 20685078

Chatoor I, Krupnick J: The role of non-specific factors in treatment outcome of psychotherapy studies. Eur Child Adolesc Psychiatry 10(suppl 1):I19–I25, 2001 11794553

Chawla AJ, Hatzmann MR, Long SR: Developing performance measures for prescription drug management. Health Care Financ Rev 22(3):71–84, 2001 25372960

Chiang CA, Jhangiani RS, Price PC: Research Methods in Psychology, 2nd Canadian Edition. BCCampus, Victoria, BC, Canada, 2015

Cohen J: Statistical Power Analysis for the Behavioral Sciences. Hillsdale, NJ, Erlbaum, 1988

Çokluk O, Kayri M: The effects of methods of imputation for missing values on the validity and reliability of scales. Educational Sciences: Theory and Practice 11(1):303–309, 2011

Cole JC: How to deal with missing data, in Best Practices in Quantitative Methods. Edited by Osborne JW. Thousand Oaks, CA, Sage, 2008, pp 214–238

Commission on Accreditation of Rehabilitation Facilities: Six Steps to Building a Performance Management System: a CARF Workbook. Tucson, AZ, CARF International, 2017. Available at: www.carf.org/performance-management-workbook. Accessed January 7, 2022.

Cousineau D, Chartier S: Outliers detection and treatment: a review. Int J Psychol Res (Medellin) 3(1):58–67, 2010

Cronbach L: Coefficient alpha and the internal structure of tests. Psychometrika 16:297–334, 1951

de Jong K, Segaar J, Ingenhoven T, et al: Adverse effects of outcome monitoring feedback in patients with personality disorders: a randomized controlled trial in day treatment and inpatient settings. J Pers Disord 32(3):393–413, 2018 28594629

Dixon L, Lieberman J: Psychiatry embraces patient-centered care. Psychiatric News, February 7, 2014. Available at: psychnews.psychiatryonline.org/doi/10.1176/appi.pn.2014.2a15. Accessed January 7, 2022.

Dodge Y: The Concise Encyclopedia of Statistics. New York, Springer, 2008

Donabedian A: Evaluating the quality of medical care. Milbank Mem Fund Q 44(3 suppl):166–206, 1966 5338568

Downey RG, King C: Missing data in Likert ratings: a comparison of replacement methods. J Gen Psychol 125(2):175–191, 1998 9935342

Dowrick C, Leydon GM, McBride A, et al: Patients' and doctors' views on depression severity questionnaires incentivized in UK quality and outcomes framework: qualitative study. BMJ 125:b663, 2009 19299474

Dunning D, Heath C, Suls JM: Flawed self-assessment: implications for health, education, and the workplace. Psychol Sci Public Interest 5(3):69–106, 2004 26158995

Eisen SV, Dickey B, Sederer LI: A self-report symptom and problem rating scale to increase inpatients' involvement in treatment. Psychiatr Serv 51(3):349–353, 2000 10686242

Eisen SV, Normand SL, Belanger AJ, et al: The Revised Behavior and Symptom Identification Scale (BASIS-R): reliability and validity. Med Care 42(12):1230–1241, 2004 15550803

Ellwood PM: Shattuck lecture—outcomes management: a technology of patient experience. N Engl J Med 318(23):1549–1556, 1988 3367968

Emilio R: What is defined in operational definitions? The case of operant psychology. Behav Philos 31:111–126, 2003

Enders C: Applied Missing Data Analysis. New York, Guilford, 2010

Epstein R: The principle of parsimony and some applications in psychology. J Mind Behav 5(2):119–130, 1984

Evans C, Margison F, Barkham M: The contribution of reliable and clinically significant change methods to evidence-based mental health. Evid Based Ment Health 1:70–72, 1998

Farooq S, Naeem F: Tackling nonadherence in psychiatric disorders: current opinion. Neuropsychiatr Dis Treat 10:1069–1077, 2014 24966677

Ferguson RJ, Robinson AB, Splaine M: Use of the reliable change index to evaluate clinical significance in SF-36 outcomes. Qual Life Res 11(6):509–516, 2002 12206571

Fiore K: Copyright issues hinder MMSE use: neurologists forced to look for alternative cognitive screening tsts. MedPage Today, June 9, 2015. Available at: www.medpagetoday.com/neurolog/dementia/52040. Accessed January 7, 2022.

Fischer R, Milfont TL: Standardization in psychological research. Int J Psychol Res (Medellin) 3(1):88–96, 2011

Folstein MF, Folstein SE, McHugh PR: "Mini-mental state": a practical method for grading the cognitive state of patients for the clinician. J Psychiatr Res 12(3):189–198, 1975 1202204

Fortney J, Sladek R, Unutzer J, et al: Fixing Behavioral Health Care in America: A National Call for Measurement-Based Care in the Delivery of Behavioral Health Services. Island Heights, NJ, The Kennedy Forum, 2015. Available at: www.thekennedyforum.org/app/uploads/2017/06/KennedyForum-MeasurementBasedCare_2.pdf. Accessed January 7, 2022.

Fortney JC, Unützer J, Wrenn G, et al: A tipping point for measurement-based care. Psychiatr Serv 68(2):179–188, 2017 27582237

Frank JD, Frank JB: Persuasion and Healing: A Comparative Study of Psychotherapy, 3rd Edition. Baltimore, MD, Johns Hopkins University Press, 1991

Frost J: Introduction to Statistics: An Intuitive Guide for Analyzing Data and Unlocking Discoveries. State College, PA, Statistics by Jim Publishing, 2019

Gamse C: Mental health comorbidity: one thing leads to another. MedPage Today, February 6, 2019. Available at: www.medpagetoday.com/resource-centers/mental-health-focus/mental-health-comorbidity-one-thing-leads-another/2408. Accessed January 7, 2022.

Garson D: Data imputation for missing values. Statistical Associated Book Series, 2015. Available at: http://www.statisticalassociates.com. Accessed May 12, 2022.

Gask L, Coventry P: Person-centred mental health care: the challenge of implementation. Epidemiol Psychiatr Sci 21(2):139–144, 2012 22789160

Gaynes BN, Rush AJ, Trivedi MH, et al: The STAR*D study: treating depression in the real world. Cleve Clin J Med 75(1):57–66, 2008 18236731

Glasgow RE: What does it mean to be pragmatic? Pragmatic methods, measures, and models to facilitate research translation. Health Educ Behav 40(3):257–265, 2013 23709579

Gonzalez J, Williams JW Jr, Noël PH, et al: Adherence to mental health treatment in a primary care clinic. J Am Board Fam Pract 18(2):87–96, 2005 15798137

Goodman JD, McKay JR, DePhillipis D: Progress monitoring in mental health and addiction treatment: a means of improving care. Prof Psychol Res Pr 44(4):231–246, 2013

Green LW: Making research relevant: if it is an evidence-based practice, where's the practice-based evidence? Fam Pract 25(suppl 1):i20–i24, 2008 18794201

Greenberg L: Emotion-Focused Therapy, 2nd Edition. Washington, DC, American Psychological Association, 2015

Greer TL, Kurian BT, Trivedi MH: Defining and measuring functional recovery from depression. CNS Drugs 24(4):267–284, 2010 20297853

Guo T, Xiang YT, Xiao L, et al: Measurement-based care versus standard care for major depression: a randomized controlled trial with blind raters. Am J Psychiatry 172(10):1004–1013, 2015 26315978

Hamel J: Case Study Methods. Qualitative Research Methods, Vol 32. Newbury Park, CA, Sage, 1993

Hannan C, Lambert MJ, Harmon C, et al: A lab test and algorithms for identifying clients at risk for treatment failure. J Clin Psychol 61(2):155–163, 2005 15609357

Harmon SC, Lambert MJ, Smart DM, et al: Enhancing outcome for potential treatment failures: therapist–client feedback and clinical support tools. Psychother Res 17(4):379–392, 2007

Hatfield D, McCullough L, Frantz SHB, et al: Do we know when our clients get worse? An investigation of therapists' ability to detect negative client change. Clin Psychol Psychother 17(1):25–32, 2010 19916162

Hawkins EJ, Lambert MJ, Vermeersch D, et al: The effects of providing patient progress information to therapists and patients. Psychother Res 14(3):308–327, 2004

Hays RD, Weech-Maldonado R, Teresi JA, et al: Commentary: copyright restrictions versus open access to survey instruments. Med Care 56(2):107–110, 2018 29256974

Heaton RK, Temkin N, Dikmen S, et al: Detecting change: a comparison of three neuropsychological methods, using normal and clinical samples. Arch Clin Neuropsychol 16(1):75–91, 2001 14590193

Hedges LV, Olkin I: Statistical Methods for Meta-Analysis. San Diego, CA, Academic Press, 1985

Henke RM, Zaslavsky AM, McGuire TG, et al: Clinical inertia in depression treatment. Med Care 47(9):959–967, 2009 19704353

Holtrop JS, Glasgow RE: Pragmatic research: an introduction for clinical practitioners. Fam Pract 37(3):424–428, 2020

Idiculla TB, Eisen SV: The BASIS-24 behavior and symptom identification scale. Integr Sci Pract 2(2):16–19, 2012

Institute of Medicine: Quality Assurance. Washington, DC, National Academies Press, 2006

Institute of Medicine: Psychological Testing in the Service of Disability Determination. Washington, DC, National Academies Press, 2015

Institute of Medicine: Crossing the Quality Chasm: A New Health System for the 21st Century. Washington, DC, National Academies Press, 2001

Jacobson NS, Truax P: Clinical significance: a statistical approach to defining meaningful change in psychotherapy research. J Consult Clin Psychol 59(1):12–19, 1991 2002127

Jacobson NS, Follette WC, Revenstorf D: Psychotherapy outcome research: methods for reporting variability and evaluating clinical significance. Behav Ther 15:336–352, 1984

Jaeschke R, Singer J, Guyatt GH: Measurement of health status: ascertaining the minimal clinically important difference. Control Clin Trials 10(4):407–415, 1989

Jerrell JM: Behavior and Symptom Identification Scale 32: sensitivity to change over time. J Behav Health Serv Res 32(3):341–346, 2005 16010189

Jette AM, Rooks D, Lachman M, et al: Home-based resistance training: predictors of participation and adherence. Gerontologist 38(4):412–421, 1998 9726128

Jin J, Sklar GE, Min Sen Oh V, et al: Factors affecting therapeutic compliance: a review from the patient's perspective. Ther Clin Risk Manag 4(1):269–286, 2008 18728716

Joint Commission: Outcome Measures Standard: CTS 03.01.09. Oakbrook Terrace, IL, The Joint Commission, 2018. Available at: www.jointcommission.org/accreditation-and-certification/health-care-settings/behavioral-health-care/outcome-measures-standard. Accessed January 7, 2022.

Jones KD: Dimensional and cross-cutting assessment in the DSM-5. J Couns Dev 90:481–487, 2012

Jones SMW, Crane PK, Simon G: A comparison of individual change using item response theory and sum scoring on the Patient Health Questionnaire-9: implications for measurement-based care. Ann Depress Anxiety 6(1):1098–1104, 2019

Jöreskog KG: A general approach to confirmatory maximum likelihood factor analysis. Psychometrika 34(2):183–202, 1969

Kang H: The prevention and handling of the missing data. Korean J Anesthesiol 64(5):402–406, 2013 23741561

Kantor LW: NIH roadmap for medical research. Alcohol Res Health 31(1):12–13, 2008 23584747

Kearney LK, Wray LO, Dollar KM, King PR: Establishing measurement-based care in integrated primary care: monitoring clinical outcomes over time. J Clin Psychol Med Settings 22(4):213–227, 2015 26645091

Kilbourne AM, Reynolds CF 3rd, Good CB, et al: How does depression influence diabetes medication adherence in older patients? Am J Geriatr Psychiatry 13(3):202–210, 2005 15728751

Kilbourne AM, Beck K, Spaeth-Rublee B, et al: Measuring and improving the quality of mental health care: a global perspective. World Psychiatry 17(1):30–38, 2018 29352529

Koh H, Sadigov S: Analyzing repeated measures data. Report No. 77, Cornell University Statistical Consulting Unit. StatNews, February 2010, pp 1–3

Kraus DR: The treatment outcome package (TOP). Integr Sci Pract 2(2):43–45, 2012

Kraus DR, Wolfe A, Castonguay LG: The outcome assistant: a kinder philosophy to the management of outcome. Psychotherapy Bulletin 41:23–31, 2006

Kroenke K, Spitzer RL, Williams JBW: The PHQ-9: validity of a brief depression severity measure. J Gen Intern Med 16(9):606–613, 2001 11556941

Lakens D: Calculating and reporting effect sizes to facilitate cumulative science: a practical primer for t-tests and ANOVAs. Front Psychol 4(863):863, 2013 24324449

Lam RW, Kennedy SH: Evidence-based strategies for achieving and sustaining full remission in depression: focus on metaanalyses. Can J Psychiatry 49(3 suppl 1):17S–26S, 2004 15147033

Lam RW, Kennedy SH: STAR*D and measurement-based care for depression: don't toss out the baby! Can J Psychiatry 60(1):6–8, 2015 25886543

Lambert MJ: Presidential address: what we have learned from a decade of research aimed at improving psychotherapy outcomes in routine care. Psychother Res 17(1):1–14, 2007

Lambert MJ: Prevention of Treatment Failure: The Use of Measuring, Monitoring, and Feedback in Clinical Practice. New York, Wiley, 2010

Lambert MJ: Maximizing psychotherapy outcome beyond evidence-based medicine. Psychother Psychosom 86(2):80–89, 2017 28183083

Lambert MJ, Burlingame GM, Umphress V, et al: The reliability and validity of the outcome questionnaire. Clin Psychol Psychother 3:249–258, 1996

Lambert MJ, Whipple JL, Hawkins EJ, et al: Is It time for clinicians to routinely track patient outcome? A meta-analysis. Clin Psychol Sci Pract 10(3):288–301, 2003

Lambert MJ, Gregersen AT, Burlingame GM: The Outcome Questionnaire 45, in The Use of Psychological Testing for Treatment Planning and Outcomes Assessment: Instruments for Adults. Edited by Maruish ME. Hillsdale, NJ, Erlbaum, 2004, pp 191–234

Lambert MJ, Harmon C, Slade K, et al: Providing feedback to psychotherapists on their patients' progress: clinical results and practice suggestions. J Clin Psychol 61(2):165–174, 2005 15609358

Lewis CC, Boyd M, Puspitasari A, et al: Implementing measurement-based care in behavioral health: a review. JAMA Psychiatry 76(3):324–335, 2019 30566197

Lieberman R, Zubrisky C, Martinez IK, et al: Using Practice-Based Evidence to Complement Evidence-Based Practice in Children's Behavioral Health. Atlanta, GA, ICF Macro, Outcomes Roundtable for Children and Families, 2010, pp 1–8

Little RJA, Rubin DB: Statistical Analysis With Missing Data. New York, Wiley, 2002

Little TD, Jorgensen TD, Lang KM, et al: On the joys of missing data. J Pediatr Psychol 39(2):151–162, 2014 23836191

Löffler W, Kilian R, Toumi M, et al: Schizophrenic patients' subjective reasons for compliance and noncompliance with neuroleptic treatment. Pharmacopsychiatry 36(3):105–112, 2003 12806568

Lucock M, Halstead J, Leach C, et al: A mixed-method investigation of patient monitoring and enhanced feedback in routine practice: barriers and facilitators. Psychother Res 25(6):633–646, 2015 26436605

Maruish ME: Outcomes assessment in health settings, in APA Handbook of Testing and Assessment in Psychology, Vol 2. Testing and Assessment in Clinical and Counseling Psychology. Edited Geisinger KF, Bracken BA, Carlson JF, et al. Washington, DC, American Psychological Association, 2013, pp 303–321

McLellan AT: Commentary on seizing the moment to improve addiction treatment. American Society of Addiction Medicine blog, August 9, 2021. Available at: www.asam.org/blog-details/article/2021/08/09/commentary-on-seizing-the-moment-to-improve-addiction-treatment. Accessed January 12, 2022.

McLellan AT, McKay JR, Forman R, et al: Reconsidering the evaluation of addiction treatment: from retrospective follow-up to concurrent recovery monitoring. Addiction 100(4):447–458, 2005 15784059

McNeeley S: Sensitive issues in surveys: reducing refusals while increasing reliability and quality of responses to sensitive survey items, in Handbook of Survey Methodology for the Social Sciences. Edited by Gideon L. New York, Springer-Verlag, 2012, pp 377–396

Melamed Y, Szor H: The therapist and the patient: coping with noncompliance. Compr Psychiatry 40(5):391–395, 1999 10509623

Michener WK: Ten simple rules for creating a good data management plan. PLOS Comput Biol 11(10):e1004525, 2015 26492633

Miller SD: The failure rate of psychotherapy. ScottDMiller.com, April 24, 2015. Available at: www.scottdmiller.com/the-failure-rate-of-psychotherapy-what-it-is-and-what-we-can-do/. Accessed January 12, 2022.

Miller SD, Duncan BL, Brown J, et al: Using formal client feedback to improve retention and outcome. Journal of Brief Therapy 5(1):5–22, 2006

Miller SD, Hubble M, Duncan B: Supershrinks: what's the secret of their success? Psychotherapy in Australia (14):14–22, 2008

Moeller SJ, Goldstein RZ: Impaired self-awareness in human addiction: deficient attribution of personal relevance. Trends Cogn Sci 18(12):635–641, 2014 25278368

Moore PJ, Sickel AE, Malat J, et al: Psychosocial factors in medical and psychological treatment avoidance: the role of the doctor-patient relationship. J Health Psychol 9(3):421–433, 2004 15117541

Morris DW, Trivedi MH: Measurement-based care for unipolar depression. Curr Psychiatry Rep 13(6):446–458, 2011 21935633

National Institute of Neurological Disorders and Stroke: User Manual for the Quality of Life in Neurological Disorders (Neuro-QoL) Measures, Version 2.0. Bethesda, MD, National Institute of Neurological Disorders and Stroke, March 2015. Available at: www.sralab.org/sites/default/files/2017-06/Neuro-QOL_User_Manual_v2_24Mar2015.pdf. Accessed January 12, 2022.

Nelson L, Proctor C, Brownie C: Responsible use of statistical methods. Ethics in Science and Engineering National Clearinghouse 301:2–26, 2000

Osbourne JW: Best Practices in Data Cleaning: A Complete Guide to Everything You Need to Do Before and After Collecting Your Data. Thousand Oaks, CA, Sage, 2013

Parent MC: Handling item-level missing data: simpler is just as good. Couns Psychol 41(4):568–600, 2013

Paronson BS, Baer DM: The visual analysis of data, and current research into the stimuli controlling it, in Single-Case Research Design and Analysis: New Directions for Psychology and Education. Edited by Kratochwill TR, Levin JR. Hillsdale, NJ, Erlbaum, 1992, pp 15–40

Perry CK, Damschroder LJ, Hemler JR, et al: Specifying and comparing implementation strategies across seven large implementation interventions: a practical application of theory. Implement Sci 14(1):32, 2019 30898133

Piriyakul M: Missing data imputation in social science research: a simple model simulation. 2006. Available at: www.research.ru.ac.th/images/ArticleMr/1501822384_Article.pdf. Accessed January 12, 2022.

Plana-Ripoll O, Pedersen CB, Holtz Y, et al: Exploring comorbidity within mental disorders among a Danish national population. JAMA Psychiatry 76(3):259–270, 2019 30649197

Powell AC, Bowman MB, Harbin HT: Reimbursement of apps for mental health: findings from interviews. JMIR Ment Health 6(8):e14724, 2019 31389336

Raney L, Lasky G, Ring J: Measurement-based care for behavioral health conditions in primary care settings: how do you know your patient improved? Health Management Associates Webinar, 2017. Available at: https://www.integratedcareconference.com/wp-content/uploads/2019/09/D6_Raney.pdf. Accessed May 7, 2022.

Richardson JTE: Eta squared and partial eta squared as measures of effect size in educational research. Educ Res Rev 6(2):135–147, 2011

Rogers JL, Nicewander WA: Thirteen ways to look at the correlation coefficient. Am Stat 42(1):59–66, 1988

Rousseeuw PJ, Hubert M: Anomaly detection by robust statistics. WIREs Data Mining and Knowledge Discovery 8(2):1–14, 2018

Rubin E, Zorumski C: The importance of insight: many psychiatric illnesses are associated with diminished insight. Psychology Today, April 7, 2016. Available at: www.psychologytoday.com/us/blog/demystifying-psychiatry/201604/the-importance-insight. Accessed January 12, 2022.

Rubin LH, Witkiewitz K, Andre JS, et al: Methods for handling missing data in the behavioral neurosciences: don't throw the baby rat out with the bath water. J Undergrad Neurosci Educ 5(2):A71–A77, 2007 23493038

Rush AJ: STAR*D: what have we learned? Am J Psychiatry 164(2):201–204, 2007 17267779

Santoyo S: A brief overview of outlier detection techniques: what are outliers and how to deal with them? Towards Data Science, September 11, 2017. Available at: towardsdatascience.com/a-brief-overview-of-outlier-detection-techniques-1e0b2c19e561. Accessed January 12, 2022.

Sapyta J, Riemer M, Bickman L: Feedback to clinicians: theory, research, and practice. J Clin Psychol 61(2):145–153, 2005 15609360

Schafer JL, Graham JW: Missing data: our view of the state of the art. Psychol Methods 7(2):147–177, 2002 12090408

Schmit EL, Balkin RS: Evaluating emerging measures in the DSM-5 for counseling practice. Prof Couns 4(3):21–31, 2014

Scott K, Lewis CC: Using measurement-based care to enhance any treatment. Cogn Behav Pract 22(1):49–59, 2015 27330267

Semahegn A, Torpey K, Manu A, et al: Psychotropic medication non-adherence and associated factors among adult patients with major psychiatric disorders: a protocol for a systematic review. Syst Rev 7(1):10–15, 2018 29357926

Shamoo AE, Resnick DB: Responsible Conduct of Research. London, Oxford University Press, 2009

Shelley PB: A Defense of Poetry. London, Edward Moxon, 1821

Shimokawa K, Lambert MJ, Smart DW: Enhancing treatment outcome of patients at risk of treatment failure: meta-analytic and mega-analytic review of a psychotherapy quality assurance system. J Consult Clin Psychol 78(3):298 311, 2010 20515206

Singh V, Rana RK, Singhal R: Analysis of repeated measurement data in the clinical trials. J Ayurveda Integr Med 4(2):77–81, 2013 23930038

Sirey JA, Bruce ML, Alexopoulos GS, et al: Stigma as a barrier to recovery: perceived stigma and patient-rated severity of illness as predictors of antidepressant drug adherence. Psychiatr Serv 52(12):1615–1620, 2001 11726752

Spikmans FJ, Brug J, Doven MM, et al: Why do diabetic patients not attend appointments with their dietitian? J Hum Nutr Diet 16(3):151–158, 2003 12753108

Stevens SS: On the theory of scales of measurement. Science 103(2684):677–680, 1946

Strupp HH: The outcome problem in psychotherapy revisited. Psychotherapy (Chic) 1:1–13, 1963 23505974

Strupp HH, Hadley SW: A tripartite model of mental health and therapeutic outcomes: with special reference to negative effects in psychotherapy. Am Psychol 32(3):187–196, 1977 848783

Substance Abuse and Mental Health Services Administration: Key Substance Use and Mental Health Indicators in the United States: Results From the 2017 National Survey on Drug Use and Health (HHS Publ No SMA 18-5068, NSDUH Series H-53). Rockville, MD, Center for Behavioral Health Statistics and Quality, Substance Abuse and Mental Health Services Administration, 2018. Available at: https://www.samhsa.gov/data. Accessed May 7, 2022.

Sullivan LM: Repeated measures. Circulation 117(9):1238–1243, 2008 18316500

Swisher AK: Practice-based evidence. Cardiopulm Phys Ther J 21(2):4, 2010 20520757

Tarlov AR, Ware JE Jr, Greenfield S, et al: The Medical Outcomes Study: an application of methods for monitoring the results of medical care. JAMA 262(7):925–930, 1989 2754793

Tavakol M, Dennick R: Making sense of Cronbach's alpha. Int J Med Educ 2:53–55, 2011 28029643

Taylor K: Paternalism, participation and partnership: the evolution of patient centeredness in the consultation. Patient Educ Couns 74(2):150–155, 2009 18930624

Thompson B: Exploratory and Confirmatory Factor Analysis: Understanding Concepts and Applications. Washington, DC, American Psychological Association, 2004

Trochim WMK: Research Methods Knowledge Base (online). April 27, 2020. Available at: conjointly.com/kb/. Accessed January 12, 2022.

Turner SM, DeMers ST, Fox HR, et al: APA's guidelines for test user qualifications: an executive summary. Am Psychol 56(12):1099–1113, 2001

Valenstein M, Adler DA, Berlant J, et al: Implementing standardized assessments in clinical care: now's the time. Psychiatr Serv 60(10):1372–1375, 2009 19797378

Van den Broeck J, Cunningham SA, Eeckels R, et al: Data cleaning: detecting, diagnosing, and editing data abnormalities. PLoS Med 2(10):e267, 2005 16138788

Vlasnik JJ, Aliotta SL, DeLor B: Medication adherence: factors influencing compliance with prescribed medication plans. Case Manager 16(2):47–51, 2005 15818344

Walfish S, McAlister B, O'Donnell P, et al: An investigation of self-assessment bias in mental health providers. Psychol Rep 110(2):639–644, 2012 22662416

Whipple JL, Lambert MJ, Vermeersch DA, et al: Improving the effects of psychotherapy: the use of early identification of treatment failure and problem-solving strategies in routine practice. J Couns Psychol 58:59–68, 2003

Widiger TA: A dimensional model of psychopathology. Psychopathology 38(4):211–214, 2005 16145277

Widiger TA, Coker LA: Mental disorders as discrete clinical conditions: dimensional versus categorical classification, in Adult Psychopathology and Diagnosis. Edited by Hersen M, Turner SM. Hoboken, NJ, Wiley, 2003, pp 3–35

Woolf SH: The meaning of translational research and why it matters. JAMA 299(2):211–213, 2008 18182604

World Health Organization: Constitution of the World Health Organization. Bull World Health Organ 80:983–984, 1946

World Health Organization: International Statistical Classification of Diseases and Related Health Problems, 10th Revision, 2nd Edition. Geneva, World Health Organization, 2004

Wray LO, Ritchie MJ, Oslin DW, et al: Enhancing implementation of measurement-based mental health care in primary care: a mixed-methods randomized effectiveness evaluation of implementation facilitation. BMC Health Serv Res 18(1):753–765, 2018 30285718

Wyrwich KW, Wolinsky FD: Identifying meaningful intra-individual change standards for health-related quality of life measures. J Eval Clin Pract 6(1):39–49, 2000 10807023

Yin RK: Case Study Research: Design and Methods, 2nd Edition. Thousand Oaks, CA, Sage, 2003

Youn SJ, Kraus DR, Castonguay LG: The treatment outcome package: facilitating practice and clinically relevant research. Psychotherapy (Chic) 49(2):115–122, 2012 22642519

Zahra D, Hedge C: The reliable change index: why isn't it more popular in academic psychology? Psychology Postgraduate Affairs Group Quarterly 76:14–19, 2010

Zerhouni EA: Translational research: moving discovery to practice. Clin Pharmacol Ther 81(1):126–128, 2007 17186011

Zettle RD: Treatment manuals, single-subject designs, and evidence-based practice: a clinical behavior analytic perspective. Psychol Rec 70(4):649–658, 2020

Zhu K, McKnight B, Stergachis A, et al: Comparison of self-report data and medical records data: results from a case-control study on prostate cancer. Int J Epidemiol 28(3):409–417, 1999 10405842

Zimek A, Filzmoser P: There and back again: outlier detection between statistical reasoning and data mining algorithms. Data Min Knowl Discov 8(6):1–37, 2018

Zimmerman M, McGlinchey JB: Depressed patients' acceptability of the use of self-administered scales to measure outcome in clinical practice. Ann Clin Psychiatry 20(3):125–129, 2008 18633738

Zimmerman M, Young D, Chelminski I, et al: Overcoming the problem of diagnostic heterogeneity in applying measurement-based care in clinical practice: the concept of psychiatric vital signs. Compr Psychiatry 53(2):117–124, 2012 21550031

Index

Page numbers printed in **boldface** type refer to tables and figures.